THE ART AND SCIENCE OF
LOW
CARBOHYDRATE
LIVING

AN EXPERT GUIDE TO MAKING THE LIFE-SAVING BENEFITS OF CARBOHYDRATE RESTRICTION SUSTAINABLE AND ENJOYABLE

Jeff S. Volek, PhD, RD
Stephen D. Phinney, MD, PhD

with contributions by:
Eric Kossoff, MD | Jacqueline Eberstein, RN | Jimmy Moore

Visit us at www.artandscienceoflowcarb.com to order additional copies.

TABLE OF CONTENTS

Section 1: Introduction

Section 2: Perspective

Section 3: Physiology

Section 4: Clinical Applications

Section 5: Guest Chapters

Section 1

INTRODUCTION

INTRODUCTION

Interesting Times

For those of us doing research on low carbohydrate diets, the last decade has given truth to the ancient Chinese curse: "may you live in interesting times." There has been a flood of scientific publications on everything from clinical studies of carbohydrate-restricted diets to underlying molecular mechanisms that explain how and why they work. And in the public domain, books and articles have critically examined the current dogma that 'carbohydrates are necessary and good, whereas dietary fats are bad'.

Meanwhile, our population just keeps on gaining and gaining: not just adults, but children as well – not just in the US, but elsewhere in the developed and developing world as well. Of course, we are not alone in being concerned about this epidemic of obesity. All sincere doctors, dietitians, scientists, and policy-makers want to turn this process around, but there is as yet no common consensus on what to do and how to do it.

There is a glimmer of hope, however. Just as we have seen the consensus change on dietary trans fats and more recently on the high fructose content in our diet, we are beginning to see movement away from diets high in carbohydrates – especially refined carbohydrates and simple sugars. But many of the mainstream experts still warn against 'going too far in the other direction', stating that there are still too many questions about the safety and efficacy of low carbohydrate diets. But is this really true? Are there still too many unanswered questions, or has this position lost traction when the flood of recent research is taken into account?

This is an important question that we feel uniquely qualified to address. Collectively, the two of us have designed, conducted, and published several dozen studies of low carbohydrate diets. These results have consistently drawn us forward to do further research because of the positive outcomes we have observed. We have counseled thousands of patients on low carbohydrate diets and tracked clinical outcomes. And as evidence of our personal convictions, both of us have chosen to follow a low carbohydrate lifestyle.

In short, we believe that the most important issues about low carbohydrate diets have now been resolved. But perhaps because we are ahead of the consensus on this, we indeed find ourselves 'living in interesting times'. Rather than being daunted by the intensity of the dialogue about low carbohydrate diets, however, we are delighted by this process, and it is this energy that has motivated us to write this book.

We ask not that you accept our position presented in this book because of our accumulated academic degrees or publications, but rather because our analysis of a broad range of information makes sense. As a place to begin, let's look at some of the obvious discords to be found in the case for maintaining the current high carbohydrate, low fat paradigm.

Five Discords

First, the 'low fat message' has been pushed in the popular media and in academia for three decades, while in this same period the prevalence of obesity in the US population has grown dramatically.

A 'low fat diet' – even one restricted in calories – is high in carbohydrate, which drives up blood insulin levels. Insulin is a hormone that drives fat into storage (i.e., into fat cells) and stimulates hunger. A low carbohydrate diet, on the other hand, allows insulin levels to remain low and fat stores to be burned in the context of reduced hunger and cravings.

Dietary saturated fat has been demonized in the media, textbooks, and in national policy; whereas published scientific data shows no connection between dietary saturated fat intake and either saturated fat levels in the body or the long term risk of heart disease.

The strongest correlation between a major dietary nutrient and blood levels of saturated fat is with dietary carbohydrate – not with saturated fat intake! On average, the more carbohydrate you eat, the higher the content of saturated fats in your blood.

And fifth, at the same time that science is increasingly defining the variability in our individual responses to diet and exercise, nutrition policy makers persist in preaching a one-size-fits-all message. For example the new Dietary Guidelines for Americans released January 31, 2011 recommends everyone consume at least 45% of their calories from carbohydrate[3]. This stands in stark contrast to the fact that their unitary edict actually matches the 'metabolic fingerprint' (i.e., the carbohydrate tolerance) of less than half of the population. Someone needs to speak up. Tantamount to pointing out the king's wardrobe failure, we can't make forward progress by moon-walking backwards.

The Unmet Need

We believe both history and science now dictate that it is time to transcend the myths and sound bites that dominate the discussion of optimum dietary fat and carbohydrate intakes. We need to get beyond the simplistic idea that all humans can and should eat the same 'perfect diet' across all phases of our life-cycle. Given the obvious metabolic diversity among humans, we need to accept dietary diversity as an important variable on achieving optimum health across the whole population.

Thus the purpose of this book – scientific evidence now supports inclusion of well-formulated low carbohydrate diets in the list of safe and sustainable dietary options to promote individual optimum health and well-being. And this is where the 'art' must join the 'science'. Just because you decide to stop eating sugar, bread, potatoes, rice and pasta doesn't mean that you have a low carbohydrate diet suitable for long-term use. That path to a well-formulated diet is more complex. In fact, understanding the 'how and why' of this formulation process takes a whole book.

Three Keys

Safety. Between the two of us, we have more than 50 years of research and clinical practice experience with low carbohydrate diets, and between us we have published a few hundred peer-reviewed papers on the topic. Much of this effort has been directed at understanding how to formulate a low carbohydrate diet for optimum safety and function. We have written this book because we are confident that a well-formulated low carbohydrate diet offers improved long-term health and well-being to people whose metabolism struggles to deal with a high carbohydrate load (aka carbohydrate intolerance).

Individual specificity. Every individual human is unique, and this variability extends to how we respond to the foods we eat. Starting two decades ago with Professor Gerald Reaven's courageous stand against the use of high carbohydrate diets in people with what we now call metabolic syndrome[4], we have become increasingly aware that some of us are 'carbohydrate intolerant'. This concept of carbohydrate intolerance is increasingly understood to be a manifestation of insulin resistance, and is associated with high blood triglycerides, high blood pressure, and in its most severe form, type-2 diabetes. These sub-groups in the population show dramatic clinical improvement when dietary carbohydrates are reduced, and thus deserve to be offered a separate path from the 'high carb, low fat' mantra promoted by national policymakers.

Sustainability (Getting Beyond 'Casual'). It is the common experience of many individuals who have naively tried a low carbohydrate diet, and also of researchers who have studied casually administered low carbohydrate diets, that normal people can't follow them for very long. But is it the low carbohydrate aspect that's at fault here, or is it specifically the casual nature of these dietary efforts that predestines most normal people to forego the long term benefits of carbohydrate restriction? The answer is that making carbohydrate restriction sustainable is complex and takes careful effort and guidance to be successful. In this book, we identify and explain many characteristics of a 'well-formulated low carbohydrate diet' suitable for long term use. In Chapter 18, for example, we summarize just the key points in this process under ten headings. Thus this topic is clearly more deserving of a book than a sound bite.

Why a Health Care Professional Should Buy this Book

Carbohydrate restriction is commonly practiced but seldom taught. Perhaps the assumption is that anyone can use common sense to figure it out (i.e., the 'casual approach'). Alternatively, those who determine the curriculum at our prestigious universities and professional schools may not believe that this topic deserves serious academic interest.

Whatever the reason, this book represents our best effort to fill the gap in information about carbohydrate restriction for health care professionals. To this end, we have attempted to walk the tight-rope of 'objectively promoting' the case for carbohydrate restriction in individuals with underlying insulin resistance or carbohydrate intolerance.

Critics will correctly state that our arguments in favor of carbohydrate restriction seem one-sided and smack of advocacy. But we ask you: what is the proper response when three decades of debate about carbohydrate restriction have been largely one-sided and driven more by cultural bias than science? Someone needs to stand up and represent the alternate view and the science that supports it.

In this effort, we have attempted to speak directly to you, the reader, rather than employ the more sterile third-person voice. Citations have been held to a minimum of the key publications in each chapter (rather than the 50-100 citations per chapter we could easily conjure up). To cover some areas where others are better versed, we also have recruited three individuals with unique experience to contribute chapters to this effort.

We have recently co-authored "The New Atkins for a New You"[5] which, while soundly based on science, is more of a step-by-step, consumer-oriented guide to following a well formulated low carbohydrate diet. This current book is functionally consistent with 'The New Atkins', but we delve deeper into how the diet works and how it can be used clinically. Thus it is more technical, but by no means do you need to be a member of MENSA to comprehend our message.

The readership of this book is not necessarily limited to healthcare professionals. Anyone with serious curiosity about nutrition and metabolism, or a desire to understand how traditional food practices can be used to improve health, will likely enjoy this book. Students and researchers in the life sciences (e.g., biochemistry, physiology, nutrition, exercise science, physical therapy, athletic training, genetics, etc.) may also find this book intriguing.

Who Ultimately Stands to Benefit from this Book?

If the people living in the United States were a pie, those who stand to benefit from restricting carbohydrate would be more than a modest slice. Currently, 2 in 3 adults qualify as overweight, and 1 in 3 is obese. In certain ethnic groups (e.g., Hispanic and Mexican American men and Black women) 4 in 5 are overweight. More than 1 in 3 adults have metabolic syndrome, 1 in 4 have impaired fasting glucose, and about 1 in 10 have type-2 diabetes. Many if not most of these people have some degree of carbohydrate intolerance and therefore would derive direct benefit from a diet low in carbohydrate. In total, this slice of the pie could represent a hundred million or more people just in the US.

The American Pie. The unremitting high prevalence of obesity, metabolic syndrome, and diabetes – all conditions that can best be described as carbohydrate intolerance - coupled with the very limited efficacy of traditional low fat diets, may be the result of forcing a square peg into a round hole. Even if you thrive on a low fat diet now, carbohydrate intolerance is increasingly prevalent as we age. Thus, over a lifetime, the majority of us may find that we are better suited to a low carbohydrate diet.

Who doesn't stand to benefit from a low carbohydrate diet? If you happen to be among the approximately 1 in 4 adults who will be blessed with the ability to thrive for a life-time on a low fat diet, consider yourself fortunate. The diet we describe here may not be appropriate for you personally, but that does not absolve you from understanding its benefits for your patients. In addition, those of us who do remain thin and healthy on a high carbohydrate diet still pay for the ill-health and lost productivity of the many who are poorly served (literally) by the 'high carb low fat' message. And while you may be metabolically blessed in being able to tolerate lots of carbohydrate now, that doesn't guarantee that this will continue as you age. It just means that you currently have more diet options than those of us with carbohydrate intolerance.

We all stand to benefit, both now and in the future, if a well-formulated low carbohydrate diet becomes an accepted option in promoting health across many sub-groups of our population. We offer this book to you in hopes that this information will broaden the options available to you and your patients in the management of carbohydrate intolerance. May we all work together towards that day when, walking down the street, we find that obesity is once again rare and no longer the norm.

Jeff Volek
Steve Phinney

Chapter 1

OVERVIEW OF LOW CARBOHYDRATE AND KETOGENIC DIETS

Historical Perspective

Who invented the low carbohydrate diet? Was it Dr. Robert Atkins' weight loss revolution in 1972? Or Wilder and Peterman's anti-seizure diet at the Mayo Clinic in the 1920's? Or perhaps Banting's pamphlet in Britain in 1863?

The answer: none of the above. But for sure, it was long, long before these recorded efforts to codify and monetize carbohydrate restriction. This does not in any way discount the contributions of these contrarian pioneers who attempted to steer us away from our sometimes fatal romance with agricultural carbohydrates. But to understand the origins of low carbohydrate metabolism and to appreciate how deeply it is rooted in our basic human physiology, we need to go back hundreds of thousands of years, if not a million or two.

Current evidence suggests that our human ancestors evolved in Africa and then spread across the globe in successive waves of migration. And while that original African ancestral group may have developed in a tropical environment where fruit and tubers could be foraged year-round, our ability as humans to migrate into barren or temperate regions depended upon our ability to survive prolonged periods of fasting, and to adapt to hunting and gathering of less carbohydrate-rich fare. And eventually, this evoked tolerance of a low carbohydrate diet allowed some humans to become highly specialized hunters and herders, living as mobile cultures in rhythm with the animals that fed them. Recent examples of these low carbohydrate nomadic cultures were the Masai herdsmen in Central Africa[6], the Bison People of the North American Great Plains[7], and the Inuit in the Arctic[8].

But long before these last low carbohydrate cultures were finally suppressed by the agricultural imperative, much of the world's populace subsisted (if not thrived) on continuous or intermittent carbohydrate restriction. For example, agricultural carbohydrates such as wheat and rye did not come north of the Alps until brought by the Romans after the time of Christ. The Irish, Scandinavians, and Russians had no agricultural carbohydrates suitable to their climate until the potato emigrated to Europe from the Andes in the 16th century AD. What this means is that many of our ancestors had little exposure to high proportions of dietary carbohydrate until 1-2 thousand years ago; and for many aboriginal cultures, their choice of a low carbohydrate lifestyle persisted to within the last few hundred years.

Now fast forward to the present. The United States is currently re-assessing a 3-decade, uncontrolled experiment in which carbohydrates were lauded and fats demonized. Concurrently we have become one of the most obese countries in the world. And across the globe, tragically, indigenous peoples with historically low carbohydrate intakes now have extremely high prevalence rates of obesity and type-2 diabetes (e.g., the Gulf States in the Middle East, Pacific Islanders, First Nations in Canada, and Australian Aborigines).

What these observations suggest is that for many humans, from an evolutionary perspective, a high carbohydrate diet is a metabolic challenge that some find difficult as early as adolescence and many fail to meet in the middle years of life. Equally apparent is that these negative effects of a high carbohydrate intake can be forestalled or reduced by vigorous exercise, high intakes of micronutrients and/or fiber from vegetables and fruit, avoidance of simple sugars, and constant energy restriction. For many

2

of us with severe obesity, metabolic syndrome, or overt type-2 diabetes, however, these 'healthy lifestyle' choices are not enough to fully counteract the negative effects of a substantial contribution of carbohydrate to our daily energy intake.

This condition, in which a collection of diseases characterized by insulin resistance are driven by consumption of a single nutrient class, deserves to be identified as "carbohydrate intolerance". And as with other single nutrient intolerances (e.g., lactose, gluten, fructose), the preferred intervention is to reduce one's dietary intake below the threshold level that produces symptoms.

What Does "Low Carbohydrate" Mean?

There are two ways to define the threshold below which you are eating a "low carbohydrate" diet. The first is defined by what you as an individual perceive – it is that level of carbohydrate intake (be it 25 grams per day or 125 grams per day) below which your signs and symptoms of carbohydrate intolerance resolve. At one end of this experiential range, someone with early signs of metabolic syndrome (e.g., high serum triglycerides and 10 extra pounds around the middle) might permanently banish these harbingers of ill-health by holding total dietary carbohydrate intake in the range of 100-125 grams per day.

At the other end of this spectrum might be a type-2 diabetic who, on a "balanced diet" providing 300 grams per day of carbohydrate, requires 2 shots of insulin plus two other oral drugs to keep fasting glucose values even marginally controlled under 150 mg/dl. For this person to achieve an optimum initial response that allows reduction (and hopefully withdrawal) of diabetic medications, clinical experience has shown that holding dietary carbohydrate at 20-to-25 grams per day is often necessary. For many type-2 diabetics, a few weeks at this level allows them to reduce or stop both insulin and oral medication while at the same time achieving better overall glucose control. A few months later, following substantial weight loss, some individuals might be able to increase daily carbohydrate intake above 50 grams per day and still maintain excellent glucose control, whereas others might need to remain below the 50 gram level to keep their type-2 diabetes in complete remission.

In either case, whether it is being able to lose weight and keep it off, or putting a frank case of type-2 diabetes into remission, how much you choose to limit your dietary carbohydrate intake should be driven by your personal experience. As a result, the amount of carbohydrate that you decide to eat might vary considerably depending on your individual metabolic condition and the level of benefit you wish to derive.

Defining 'Nutritional Ketosis'

The second way to define 'low carbohydrate' is physiologic – specifically that level below which there is a fundamental shift in your body's fuel homeostasis (i.e., energy regulation) away from glucose as a primary fuel. This shift is the adaptation of the body's hormonal set and inter-organ fuel exchange to allow most of your daily energy needs to be met by fat, either directly as fatty acids or indirectly by ketone bodies made from fat. This process, which is discussed more fully in Chapter 7, begins for most adults when total carbohydrate is restricted to less than 60 grams per day along with a moderate intake of protein. After a few weeks at this level, the primary serum 'ketone' (beta-hydroxybutyrate, or B-OHB), rises above 0.5 millimolar (mM). At this ketone level, which is 10-fold higher than that in someone with a daily intake of 300 grams of carbohydrate, the brain begins to derive a substantial portion of its energy needs from B-OHB, resulting in a commensurate reduced need for glucose.

With further restriction of carbohydrate below 50 grams per day, the serum B-OHB rises in response to reduced insulin secretion. However, because dietary protein prompts some insulin release, and serum B-OHB itself stimulates insulin release by the pancreas (albeit subtly), adults eating 20 grams of carbohydrate and 75-150 grams per day of protein rarely run serum B-OHB levels above 3 mM. This is in contrast to the response to total starvation (i.e., no dietary carbs or protein) where the serum B-OHB levels run as high as 5 mM.

This 10-fold range of serum ketones, from 0.5 to 5 mM, is your body's normal physiological response to varying degrees of dietary carbohydrate and protein restriction. This response range is called 'nutritional ketosis', and is associated with metabolic adaptations allowing your body to maintain a stable state of inter-organ fuel homeostasis. This process is dependent on an adequate, albeit minimal, ability of the pancreas to produce insulin in response to dietary protein and serum ketones, thus maintaining serum B-OHB in the range where it replaces much of your body's (and your brain's) need for glucose without distorting whole-body acid-base balance.

Nutritional ketosis is by definition a benign metabolic state that gives human metabolism the flexibility to deal with famine or major shifts in available dietary fuels. By contrast, 'diabetic ketoacidosis' is an unstable and dangerous condition that occurs when there is inadequate pancreatic insulin response to regulate serum B-OHB. This occurs only in type-1 diabetics or in late stage type-2 diabetes with advanced pancreatic burnout. In this setting of deficient insulin, when exogenous insulin is withheld, serum B-OHB levels reach the 15-25 mM range – 5-to-10-fold higher than the levels characteristic of nutritional ketosis.

Unfortunately, among the general public and even many health care professionals as well, these two distinct metabolic states tend to be confused one for another. Understanding how different they are is key to being able to capture the many benefits of nutritional ketosis while avoiding the risks in that very small minority of the population subject to developing diabetic ketoacidosis. To this end, a full chapter later in this book is devoted to the clinical use of carbohydrate restriction in diabetes.

Utility and Sustainability of Carbohydrate Restriction

Up until 150 years ago, the apparent motivation for humans to eat a low carbohydrate diet was because that was what their regional environment provided. For example, absent wild orchards and fields of waving grain, the Inuit had little choice other than meat and fat from the arctic tundra and the sea. However, some cultures with long experience and apparent choice attempted to actively defend their low carbohydrate lifestyle. Examples of this included the Bison People of the North American Great Plains, who maintained their nomadic existence until the bison were virtually exterminated, and the Masai of East Africa who still avoided vegetable foods (against the vigorous advice of the British) into the 1930s. Manifestly, for these cultures, not only were their low carbohydrate dietary practices sustainable – allowing them to survive and reproduce for hundreds of generations under difficult environmental conditions – they regarded their diet of animal products as preferable to an agricultural lifestyle, despite the latter having been available to them.

In the 1920s, carbohydrate restriction was employed in mainstream medical practice in the management of diabetes and in the treatment of seizures. In both of these clinical situations, as there was no other effective treatment, these dietary interventions were sustained by individual patients for years. With the advent of insulin for diabetes and anti-seizure drugs like diphenyl-hydantoin (Dilantin), these dietary interventions began to fall out of favor. However now that the practical limitations and side effects of modern pharmaceutical therapy are becoming recognized, the wheel may be again turning.

One of the perceived limitations of modern low carbohydrate diets is that they have become stigmatized as extreme and thus necessarily limited to temporary use. Adding to this sense of transience, most popular diet books promoting carbohydrate restriction have effectively only described an initial energy restricted phase to promote weight loss. So what does the reader do after 3 months eating 1400 kcal/day with a 30 lb weight loss? No healthy adult over 5 feet tall achieves energy balance on 1400 kcal per day, so the transition from weight loss to long-term weight maintenance necessarily means adding back food. But how much, and from what foods? Carbohydrates? Protein? Fat?

It is a primary hypothesis (if not principle) of this book that a low carbohydrate diet that is sustainable in the long term (e.g., for the management of type-2 diabetes, seizures, or severe obesity) necessarily contains an appropriate fat content in its weight maintenance phase. Thus, if a book promoting a low carb diet does not contain practical instruction and recipes promoting the inclusion of fat in its maintenance diet, it is not likely to result in much long-term success among its readers. To this end, later chapters in this book will describe the physiology of fuel partitioning, clinical use of low carbohydrate and ketogenic diets, plus two full chapters and a week's worth of menus addressing the practicalities of preparing and consuming a maintenance diet that is rich in fat.

Recent and Future Research

The last decade has seen a dramatic increase in the volume of research publication on the topic of carbohydrate restriction. Multiple randomized, controlled trials (RCTs) have been performed comparing a variety of other diets to carbohydrate restriction. Many of these have demonstrated clear advantages in favor of low carbohydrate and ketogenic diets. However, the interpretation of these studies is sometimes clouded by reticence of authors or editors to give them due credit or by pitfalls in research methodology. The pros and cons of this recent body of research are addressed throughout this book. In addition, multiple contributing authors provide their insights on topics pertinent to the range of effects and benefits of carbohydrate restriction.

Section 2

PERSPECTIVE

Chapter 2

LOW CARBOHYDRATE LESSONS FROM ABORIGINAL CULTURES

Introduction and Caveat

Human experience with low carbohydrate diets began when this planet's first primates chased down and killed some unfortunate but succulent animal and then could not find any nearby wild tubers to serve with the meat. Rather than starve, they probably decided with some reluctance to accept the indignity of a meal consisting of just meat and fat. That event likely occurred well over 2 million years ago, after which our ancestors stumbled about in the dietary darkness until the development of modern agriculture brought us a dependable supply of carbohydrates starting maybe 8000 years ago. And in some remote corners of the earth, the arrival of agricultural carbohydrate has only occurred within the last century. But for almost all of our ancestors, in the intervening 2 million years, humans had to figure out how to make do with just meat and fat as their primary sources of dietary energy.

Getting a low carbohydrate diet "right" is not as simple as just avoiding sugars and starches. One has to decide how much and what sources of protein and fats to seek out. Then comes developing methods to prepare them and maybe even to store them. Along with enough energy and protein, our intrepid ancestors also had to figure out how to get their minimum requirement for minerals and vitamins to reach adulthood and re-produce. Given the obvious fact that at least some of them survived this gauntlet, there had to have been pockets of people who figured it all out. But maybe it's not all that much of a surprise. After all, they had around 2 million years of trial and error to do so.

Practically speaking, what this means is that most of the important principles of carbohydrate-restricted diets were discovered eons ago. Unfortunately, those people holding this information were usually not literate, so this dietary information was never carved in stone and thus tended to die with them, and with their cultures. Equally unfortunate, the often literate people whose contact brought agricultural foods to the Earth's last remaining hunting cultures were often less than accurate reporters of the pre-contact cultures they were observing. Thus what we do 'know' of the dietary practices of aboriginal hunting peoples was seen through the lens of cultural bias. This necessitates an important caveat: beware of ethno-centric interpretation of aboriginal behaviors.

It is a normal human tendency to interpret the behavior of others through the lens of our own cultural practices. Nomadic people, for example, are often viewed as unsettled or uncivilized because they do not build and maintain permanent houses or villages. As for dietary practices, people who cannot imagine themselves living without copious dietary carbohydrate (our daily bread) will tend to look for the hidden dietary carbohydrate sources, however improbable, in the diets of hunters.

That said, however, it is the hypothesis of this chapter that not all that is written about the diets of hunters and nomadic shepherds is incorrect, and when assessed against a modern understanding of metabolism, much of the bias and mythology can be peeled away, leaving a sparse but useful truth.

The reason we should be motivated to undertake this effort is the inescapable conclusion that the dietary path down which industrialized cultures have wandered this last century is clearly not leading us to health and wellbeing. And to better understand where we should be going, perhaps it might help to thoughtfully examine where we have been.

Seeking Credible Reporters

It is therefore useful to exercise caution when evaluating reports of observers, even scientifically trained ones, who regard their nomadic objects of study as culturally inferior (or as savages, for that matter). The better observers are those who lived among, ate the food, and traveled with the hunting or herding cultures they were studying. Such individuals included George Catlin among the Plains Indian[7], John Rae[9], Frederick Schwatka[10], and Vilhjalmur Stefansson among the Inuit[8], plus John Orr and J.L.Gilks among the Masai[6].

All of these observers comment on the esteem that hunting and herding peoples held for fat. Buffalo hunted in the fall, fattened from a summer of grazing, were used by the Plains Indian to make pemmican (i.e., a mixture of dried meat and hot fat that cools to become a stable block when sealed in a raw-hide sack). Caribou were similarly hunted in the fall along their migration routes from the tundra back to the forests, when the rapidly dropping temperature allowed the meat and fat to be stored frozen in caches for winter use. Along the Pacific Coast, vast quantities of a smelt-like fish (called the oolichan) were harvested, processed, and the 'grease' stored in cedar boxes for year-around use and for trade with inland bands.

What is generally lacking, however, is accurate quantitative information on the proportions of fat, protein, and carbohydrate eaten by these aboriginal cultures prior to European contact. We do have Orr and Gilks report[6] of the daily food intake of a Masai warrior-class male: 1.2 kg of meat, 2 liters of milk, and 50 ml of blood. But we don't know the fat contents of the meat and milk, which can vary greatly on the cut of the meat, the preparation of the cattle before slaughter, and the amount of cream included in the milk.

Finding Credible Dietary Quantitation

Perhaps our best transducer of the pre-contact Inuit diet is Stefansson during his one-year of closely monitored dietary intake while participating in the Bellevue experiment (see sidebar). With both his reputation and well-being riding on the outcome of this experiment, it is a good assumption that he would have earnestly attempted to reproduce those dietary practices of the Inuit which had previously sustained him for a decade in the Arctic. The published results of this experiment tell us that Stefansson ate 15% of his daily energy as protein, over 80% as fat, and a few percent as carbohydrate (from glycogen naturally found in the meat)[11].

Putting His Life on the Line: Stefansson's Inuit Diet Experiment

In 1907, a Harvard-trained Canadian anthropologist went into the Canadian Arctic to study the Inuit culture. Whether by chance or design, he spent his first Arctic winter living among the native people of the region without any external food supply. Eight months later, he emerged speaking their language and empowered by the fact that he could live well off the available food of the region.

A decade later, Vilhjalmur Stefansson left the Arctic, having traveled where no person of European origin had gone before, sometimes for two years without any resupply. Upon his return to 'civilization', he wrote copiously about his experience among 'The People' (which is what "Inuit" means in their language).

Unfortunately for Stefansson, the decade between 1915 and 1925 was the era of vitamin discovery – the period in which scientific nutrition hit its stride. Suddenly, we had scientists to tell us what was good for us, replacing grandmothers and cultural wisdom. And scientists now said that all humans needed fruit and vegetables to prevent deficiency diseases like scurvy and beriberi.

To the newly-minted nutritionists of the 1920s, Stefansson became the proverbial buck wearing a bulls-eye. To salvage his reputation, he consented (along with an Arctic explorer colleague) to reproduce his Inuit diet under continuous observation in Bellevue Hospital in New York City. After a year, he and his colleague emerged hale and hearty, much to the disappointment of the scientists in charge.

What Stefansson's experience (and many other subsequent studies) demonstrated was that dietary carbohydrate is nutritionally superfluous in the context of a well-formulated low carbohydrate diet.

Furthermore, the fact that aboriginal pemmican (not the condiment version loaded with nuts and berries to suit European tastes) provided about 75% of its energy from fat necessarily leads us away from the common misconception that hunters' diets were high in protein. Even the Masai dietary data provided by Orr and Gilks (if we use modern meat and milk composition data) suggest that they ate about 30% of energy as protein and 70% as fat. Thus we have a range for the proportion of fat in culturally evolved hunting and herding diets from 70% to more than 80% of daily energy intake.

There are, of course, extensive published data that dispute these proportions. Analyses of food waste from cave floors and village middens (mounds of discarded household waste) often suggests higher protein intakes, leading some to contend that a 'typical hunter-gatherer' ate 40-50% of his energy as protein, 20% as carbohydrates, and only 40% or so as fat. However there are a number of problems with getting good quantitative information by this method. For example, it does not allow us to know which parts of the food were treasured, which discarded, and what parts were fed to the dogs.

Among the Inuit, when a seal or caribou was killed, the fat was saved for human consumption (or lamp fuel) and the leaner parts were given to the dogs (or any gullible 'white guys' in the party). Farther to the south, when a spring buffalo (i.e., one that had yet to rebuild body fat reserves after the winter) was killed on the Great Plains, the humans ate the tongue, liver, and marrow. These tissues tended to retain their fat content even during periods of privation. The lean meat was either dried (to serve as an emergency food source) or fed to the dogs. This differential partitioning of the kill actually makes a lot of sense, as a dog's metabolism is much more tolerant of a high protein intake than is that of a human. But how this was done in a quantitative sense cannot be divined by examining animal bones and sea shells in village trash heaps (i.e., 'middens'). So how does one say in Latin *"beware of garbage dump science"*?

Another limitation of studying these refuse middens is that they only occur adjacent to long term sites of habitation, such as towns or villages. However, some of the most highly evolved hunting societies were nomadic. If you spend most of your year on the prairie following the migration of the buffalo, you are not going to spend enough time in one site to create a midden. And if you manufacture pemmican at multiple sites along your migration path and return with it every year to a protected winter camp, then nothing you discard in an adjacent dump will inform the modern investigator that much of your diet consisted of fat that was harvested elsewhere before coming into that camp.

Similar concerns would apply to shell middens found on the British Columbia coast and elsewhere. These imply a high intake of shellfish protein. However if fresh shellfish harvested in the fall and winter are dipped in oolichan grease transported from a distant spring oolichan camp, that component of the diet would not be appreciated by examining the midden at the winter camp. So here again, standard anthropological techniques used to analyze the composition of aboriginal hunting and fishing diets may mislead us as to the diet's fat content, particularly if the investigator comes to the topic with the preconception that such diets were high in protein.

Type of Fat Consumed

There is copious evidence that established hunting societies were selective of the types of fat that they acquired and ate. These choices seem to have been made for a number of reasons, including the shelf-life of specific fats (i.e., storability) as well as the nutritional properties of the different types of fat available. In the same way that herding societies processed milk to produce butter and cheese for long-term storage, hunters developed methods to process and store fats to tide them through lean periods in the hunting cycle.

Pemmican was a staple of the bison people living on the Great Plains of North America. From Texas to the Canadian Prairie Provinces, teepees were erected next to a kill, the fat cut away and saved as the meat was dried in the sun or over a slow fire. A few days later, as their dogs consumed the last unwanted bits of cartilage and sinew, these people struck camp and departed with full stomachs and 100-200 pounds of reserve food. At those times when a fresh kill evaded them, an individual could remain healthy and happy on a pound of pemmican per day. So when hunting was good and the buffalo fat, families could process and transport with them a couple of months' food supply.

While pemmican was obviously produced on the basis of availability, the priority of its consumption was based upon its physical properties. Late summer and fall pemmican was richer in saturated fats, making it firmer and thus was more resistant to melting and rancidity. This pemmican could be held in reserve for a year or two without going bad. In contrast, winter pemmican, made with body fat that was richer in polyunsaturates, tended to be 'softer' and was more prone to rancidity. So these lots got consumed sooner rather than later.

It was this summer pemmican that became a standard trade item of the upper Midwest in the 18th and 19th centuries as the Canadian Northwest and Hudson's Bay Companies came to dominate the regional fur trade. Pemmican fueled the transport of furs out of the Canadian interior in freight canoes, paddled by voyageurs who had no time to stop and hunt as they pushed a total of 3000 miles up the St. Lawrence River and Great Lakes and back in a single season. But long before the Europeans came, archeological evidence tells us that the aboriginal people of the Great Plains were already trading pemmican to their distant neighbors for pipestone, tobacco, flint, beaver, ermine, and even seashells.

But the fat most valued and most extensively traded in aboriginal North America was extracted from an obscure little fish that appeared for just a week along the North Pacific coast every year in March (until recently). From the Klamath River in Northern California to the Aleutians, an icon of the aboriginal people in the region was the oolichan (aka eulachon or candlefish). This little forager of the Pacific came into inlets and estuaries every spring in vast numbers, where for 10 millennia the aboriginal people would gather in anticipation of its return.

There were three major sources of fish fat available to the aboriginal everyman in this region: salmon, eel, and oolichan. Hunting larger game like whale, sea lion, and seal required access to the sea and the use of sea-going canoes. Some but not all coastal peoples had the technology to construct these large boats. But if you were shore-bound, the salmon, eel, and particularly the oolichan came to you – dependably, year after year, century after century. Dependability you could build a culture on.

The oolichan is up to 20% fat by weight. When you hang it out to dry, it becomes a dry stick that you can light like a candle in your winter lodge so you can see in the dark – thus its name 'candlefish'. But more importantly, a ton of fresh fish harvested in March yields up to 400 pounds of fat you can extract, store in cedar boxes, and eat throughout the year.

Why process and store oolichan grease? Because not only was it available – it was unique! Unlike the oil from seal, whale, and salmon, oolichan fat is very low in polyunsaturates (both omega-3 and omega-6)[12]. Its primary fatty acids are mono-unsaturated, much like olive oil. That plus its content of saturated fats makes it a semi-solid at 'room temperature', so it was much more easily stored and transported in the bent-wood cedar boxes crafted for this purpose by local artisans.

Archeological evidence indicates that oolichan 'grease' was produced along the North Pacific coast by the ton, much of which was carried inland for trading purposes along established 'grease trails'. In exchange, the coastal people got beaver pelts, flint, copper, and dried moose meat from inland sources. Some of these grease trails extended hundreds of miles into the interior, and they were used to transport this unique dietary staple inland for thousands of years.

So why might this be? Why wait around for a school of little fish when harpooning a single whale or a few sea lions gives you the same amount of fat? The answer is found in lipid chemistry – the more double bonds you have in a given amount of fat, the sooner it goes rancid. Rancidity occurs when oxygen molecules are added to the fat, changing the taste and destroying its nutritional value. The human nose identifies rancid fat as offensive. And seal, whale, and most fish oils go rancid within a few weeks unless refrigerated or stored in airtight containers, whereas oolichan grease (like olive oil) can be stored for a year or more without going rancid.

Which Came First? Oolichan Grease or Olive Oil.

In a recent conversation with Bill Moore, a local fisherman of the Niska'a Band in Greenville (Laxgalts'ap), British Columbia, one of us suggested that oolichan grease is like olive oil from the sea. Bill thought for a moment and then responded: "we have been harvesting the oolichan for 9000 years, which is a lot longer than people have grown olives; so maybe we should think of olive oil as oolichan grease from the land."

But there's another reason why oolichan grease was wildly popular in the pre-contact Pacific Northwest. Again, this can be explained in part by simple chemistry. The human body stores fat for reserve energy to sustain itself if there is nothing else to eat, and our bodies seem to favor the storage of monounsaturates over other classes of fatty acids. Monounsaturates, along with saturates, appear to be what our cells want to burn when they are adapted to burning mostly fat. Oolichan grease is rich in monounsaturates, and thus is more like human fat than anything else in the region. Thus oolichan grease appears to have an ideal fat composition for humans who consume a diet appropriately rich in fat. Somehow, without the benefit of modern chemistry or nutritionists to tell them what to do, a diverse collection of peoples inhabiting 3000 miles of the Pacific coastline of North America discovered this, and built their cultures and a regional trade economy around this one source of fat.

Salt

Whole books have been written about the history of salt. Wars were fought over access to salt. Roman soldiers were often paid with a measure of salt, hence the origin of the English word 'salary'. Hunters and their prey, herders and their cattle, all shaped their actions and habits around access to salt. The reason, of course, is that salt (sodium) is necessary for life.

Humans did not need to know chemistry to understand the value of salt. Salt deprivation leads to lightheadedness, fatigue, headache, and malaise. Aboriginal cultures could figure out that if they drank from one spring, they began to feel lousy, but if they drank from that other one, they'd feel OK. The Inuit knew which ice to melt for water to boil their meat. Sea ice loses its salt content with age. Fresh ice had too much salt, fresh snow had none, whereas older sea ice was just right.

Inland hunters followed their prey to salt licks and salt springs. These waters were prized for cooking, and some cultures learned to dry these waters to make dry salt. But the universal dependable source of salt for inland hunters and herders alike was blood. Blood was collected from freshly killed animals using the emptied stomach as a container, whether from a bison on the Great Plains or from caribou or muskox on the tundra. A liter of whole blood contains about 2 grams of sodium, so 500 ml per day would ward off acute symptoms of salt depletion.

Among the Masai living in hot inland Kenya, the consumption of blood was a staple of their culture (along with meat and milk). Even in the 1920's, long after British trade had provided them access to dry salt, the Masai still bled their cattle to provide each hunter with a token 50 ml of blood per day[6]. Given another century of perspective, perhaps the perjorative phrase misrepresenting many aboriginal cultures as 'bloodthirsty savages' might better be replaced by the phrase 'bloodthirsty savants'.

Today we 'know' that too much salt is bad for us, so why this long discussion of a discredited nutrient? The short answer is that the amount of carbohydrate in our diet changes our need for salt. High carbohydrate diets make the kidneys retain salt, whereas a low carbohydrate intake increases sodium excretion by the kidney (called 'the natriuresis of fasting'). Hunting cultures seemed to understand this, and thus their highly evolved practices of finding sodium and consuming enough of it to maintain health and well-being.

Summary

The last few decades have yielded a lot of scientific knowledge about low carbohydrate diets, but in the few thousand millennia preceding the development of modern science, our hunting and herding ancestors solved the practical problems needed to live and function well with a minimal carbohydrate intake. They didn't need to know how it worked, just that it did. Successful dietary practices were integrated into their cultures and passed along across generations.

But as these traditional cultures were overwhelmed and replaced by agriculture, much of this hard won knowledge has been lost. This is unfortunate, given the potential value that low carbohydrate diets offer us, particularly in the management of diseases associated with insulin resistance. So let us summarize three lessons plucked from a few of these cultures.

1. First, a well formulated low carbohydrate diet is moderate in protein and higher in fat. People attempting to follow a low carbohydrate diet that is also low in fat will find it unpleasant if not unhealthy and difficult to sustain. Aboriginal cultures knew that the body prefers fat over protein as fuel.

2. Second, the type of fat eaten when most of your energy comes from fat is important. If you are a hunter getting 70-80% of your energy from fat, your dietary fat composition needs to be different from what you would consume if you were a subsistence farmer eating mostly carbohydrates with just 15% of your energy as fat. When fat is used for fuel, the body prefers that the majority of it be provided as mono-unsaturates and saturates. On a low carbohydrate diet appropriately rich in fat, even if only a small proportion of your fat is polyunsaturated, this small fraction times the total amount will still provide enough grams of the essential fatty acids. Because they function like vitamins rather than fuel, for the essential

21

fatty acids, it's all about dose, not percent. And for the omega-6 fats in particular, more is not necessarily better. (See Chapter 9, Effects of Carbohydrate Restriction on Fatty Acid Metabolism)

3. Third, the body's metabolism of salt is uniquely different when one is adapted to a low carbohydrate diet. Salt and water are more efficiently excreted, which is a good thing as long as you maintain an adequate minimum sodium intake. Ignore this lesson and you are likely to suffer the completely avoidable problems of headache, fatigue, weakness, and constipation – maladies that any Inuit healer would have promptly resolved by giving you a bowl of blood soup, or meat broth made with sea ice of the proper age.

Chapter 3

THE "MODERN" HISTORY OF CARBOHYDRATE RESTRICTION

Introduction

In the realm of practical nutrition, by which we mean what people actually eat day in and day out, there is little new in the world. The spate of clinical studies in the last 10 years comparing the effects of low fat versus low carbohydrate diets on body weight and blood lipids merely echo much of the work of scientists spanning the last two centuries. This, in combination with the empirical experience of aboriginal cultures that lived by hunting or herding (as discussed in the preceding chapter), offers us a rich background upon which to judge the current turmoil surrounding dietary carbohydrate.

Stepping back a bit from the current fray, the fact that there is turmoil surrounding the relative roles of dietary fats and carbohydrates is itself rather surprising. After all, modern organic chemistry cut its teeth on nutrient composition (along with dyes and petrochemicals) starting in the mid 1800s. Now, one and a half centuries later, we should have universal agreement on the definitive information telling us what is best for humans to eat. For example, how could the carbohydrate-fat controversy not be resolved after we paid $700 million to perform the Women's Health Initiative (an assessment of both a low fat diet and hormone replacement) on 50,000 women completed in 2006?

The explanation for the ongoing carbohydrate-fat controversy is fascinatingly complex, and not surprisingly, it probably has more to do with politics and egos than with science per se. At the crux of our current diet dilemma is the 1977 McGovern Committee's publication **Dietary Goals for the United States**. This document, primarily produced by a group of lawyers and journalists serving on McGovern staff, was influenced more by personal opinion than by the technical expertise in the field. While revised guidelines were published by the USDA in 1980, they still exhorted Americans to: "Avoid Too Much Fat, Saturated Fat, and Cholesterol".

In response to this less-than-scientifically-rigorous process, in that same year the Food and Nutrition Board of the National Academy of Sciences released a competing document **Toward Healthful Diets** that avoided recommendations on fat and cholesterol intakes, focusing instead on maintaining a healthy body weight. Rather than being welcomed into a meaningful discussion, the Food and Nutrition Board's chairperson at the time, Dr. Philip Handler, was vigorously pressured to toe the party line. In an eloquently understated response, giving the following testimony before a congressional committee in 1980, Dr Handler did...and then courageously did not...acquiesce:

> *However tenuous the linkage, however disappointing the various intervention trials, it still seems prudent to propose to the American public that we not only maintain reasonable weights for our height, body structure and age, but also reduce our dietary fat intakes significantly, and keep cholesterol intake to a minimum. And, conceivably, you might conclude that it is proper for the federal government to so recommend.*
>
> *On the other hand, you may instead argue: What right has the federal government to propose that the American people conduct a vast nutritional experiment, with them-*

selves as subjects, on the strength of so very little evidence that it will do them any good?

Mr. Chairman, resolution of this dilemma turns on a value judgment. The dilemma so posed is not a scientific question; it is a question of ethics, morals, politics. Those who argue either position strongly are expressing their values; they are not making scientific judgments.

Now, with the three intervening decades lending acuity to our hindsight, Dr. Handler's cautionary position appears to have been precisely correct. Understanding how he and his fellow scientists came to be ignored, and how as a result our population has developed more obesity, diabetes, and many forms of cancer over the last 30 years, is an important lesson that would serve us well to study.

One of the clearer voices in the recent dialogue about low carbohydrate diets is that of Gary Taubes. A renowned (and some might say, courageous) science writer, Taubes weighed in on the topic with a New York Times Magazine article entitled "What If It's Been A Big Fat Lie?" in June 2002. Taubes has subsequently presented in depth analyses of these dietary controversies in two books - Good Calories, Bad Calories[13] and Why We Get Fat [14]. We highly recommend reading these definitive and carefully referenced books for the full story, but the next few pages will touch on some key points presented by Taubes in his chronicle of the dietary carbohydrate-fat controversy

Banting's *Letter on Corpulence*

In 1862, a retired British undertaker named William Banting was struggling to contain his weight. All of the usual nostrums of the Victorian medical establishment – exercise, calorie restriction, purgatives – failed to work.

As an aside, it is interesting how little has changed since the mid-1800's, Most doctors still prescribe exercise and calorie restriction, and the most popular drug in use (Orlistat, aka Xenocal or Alli) acts by blocking intestinal fat absorption (i.e., it's a purgative).

Eventually he consulted a surgeon named William Harvey who had studied in Paris.

At that time on the Continent there was interest in diets limited in sugars and starches, so Harvey prescribed such a diet for William Banting.

Within a year, Banting had lost 50 pounds while suffering none of the unpleasant side effects of his other weight loss attempts. He was so pleased with his success on Harvey's diet that he published a 16-page pamphlet describing this diet and its effects. It sold well not only in Britain but in the US as well, and it was also translated into multiple other languages. Within a few years, 'to bant' became a verb synonymous with dieting.

The diet Harvey prescribed for Banting consisted of meat, fish, and poultry, no limitation on animal and dairy fats, small portions of low sugar fruits, and even a few bits of toast. Otherwise no sugars, sweets, or starches were allowed. Beer, which is rich in carbs, was forbidden, but wine and distilled spirits were allowed if not encouraged. In addition to initially acknowledging Harvey, later editions of Banting's pamphlet also acknowledged the work of the French physicians who had influenced Harvey.

Thus the diet promoted by Banting was not invented by this undertaker out of thin air but rather had its roots in the mainstream medicine of its day. However, its rapid rise to popular use caused concerns among the more conservative medical leaders of the day, who spoke out against it, at first claiming that it offered nothing new and then warning (without any scientific evidence) that it could be dangerous. The public was obviously not convinced by this pushback, however, as the Banting regimen and similar diets remained popular well into the 20th century, and it had support from some in the medical community as well. Sir William Osler, the renowned Johns Hopkins physician and one of the fathers of mainstream medicine in the US, commented favorably on Banting's regimen in his iconic textbook **The Principles and Practice of Medicine** in 1892.

The Eisenhower Opportunity

In 1955, President Dwight Eisenhower suffered a heart attack, after which his next 4 years in office were spent under an intense media spotlight. Despite having a completely normal serum cholesterol level and normal body weight at the time of his myocardial infarction, he was convinced by his medical advisors that he had to reduce his intake of fat and cholesterol. Soldiers, even generals like Eisenhower, are used to taking orders, so he did as he was told. In response, to everyone's dismay, both his weight and blood cholesterol level went up rather than down. So he redoubled his dietary restrictions and obsessed over his blood test results. It was a classic case of 'doing better but feeling worse'.

But that didn't stop the public health experts of the time, like Professor Ancel Keys of the University of Minnesota, from taking this opportunity to promote a low fat, low cholesterol diet for the whole nation. The rationale was that the United States was suffering from an epidemic of heart disease (which was anything but a proven fact), and something had to be done to contain it. And since animal fats contained cholesterol, and arterial plaques contained cholesterol, connecting these dots was an easy story to sell.

Meanwhile the research community set about trying to pour solid concrete under this dietary house of cards. In the 1970s, two massive studies were started on men with high blood cholesterol levels. The first, called the Multiple Risk Factor Intervention Trial (MRFIT) used a very low fat diet, exercise, blood pressure control and smoking cessation to try and reduce heart attack risk[15]. The second, the Lipid Research Clinics (LRC) study, tested the combination of a low fat diet plus the cholesterol lowering drug cholestyramine[16].

Close to a decade later, the results of these studies were tallied. For the MRFIT subjects who did everything they were told, there was a slight <u>increase</u> in the death rate compared to those in the placebo group who did nothing at all. In the LRC study, the cholesterol lowering drug slightly reduced the number of heart attacks compared to the placebo group, but overall mortality in the two groups was not significantly different. Specifically, out of 1800 men in each group, 68 died in the treatment group and 71 in the placebo group.

Ignoring the fact that the MRFIT study got the opposite result from what they had predicted, and that the effect of the LRC study on overall mortality was insignificant, the advocates of the dietary fat/cholesterol hypothesis set to work selling the United States Government and people on the idea that eating less fat and cholesterol was good for their health. And in the process, cautionary voices such as Dr. Philip Handler (quoted above) were steam-rolled by a vocal group of anti-fat advocates.

As for President Eisenhower, in the 13 years after his first heart attack, he followed his doctor's orders with military precision. Despite sticking closely to a very low fat, high carbohydrate diet, he suffered from persistent digestive problems and 6 more heart attacks, the last of which killed him in 1969.

Robert C. Atkins: a Revolution Built upon Historical Rock

In the early 1960s, Dr. Robert C. Atkins, a cardiologist trained at Cornell Medical College and practicing in New York City, put himself on a low carbohydrate diet and easily lost weight that he previously had struggled to lose. Recommending this diet to others, he observed that they too were successful at losing. Soon he had built a sizeable clinical practice in which he refined the use of dietary carbohydrate restriction as a therapeutic tool.

In retrospect, Dr. Atkins' timing could have been better. The 1970s was probably not the best time to be extolling the virtues of very low carbohydrate diets. That's because the mainstream nutrition consensus led by Dr. Frederick Stare at Harvard and Dr. Theodore Van Itallie at Columbia increasingly portrayed low carbohydrate diets as dangerously high in fat. To do so, they needed to ignore considerable contemporary work by Dr. John Yudkin of Queen's College in London and Dr. Charlotte Young at

Cornell (whose research possibly influenced Dr. Atkins, who was trained at Cornell). These and other respected scientists had demonstrated safe and rapid weight loss with reduced hunger by prescribing low carbohydrate diets unrestricted in fat. But like Dr. Handler, these scientifically credible voices were no match for Drs. Stare and Van Itallie. They too were steam-rolled or ignored.

Given this hostile academic climate, being in private practice was clearly an asset for Dr. Atkins. Unlike university faculty who need to get grants funded and papers published, Atkins was not dependent upon consensus committees (the peer-review system used by the NIH) for research grants or on journal editors who decided which papers to accept or reject. As a result, he was less inhibited than his academic contemporaries and thus less prone to being steam-rolled. And, although Dr. Atkins was branded a heretic and quack by his contemporary medical peers, his books nonetheless reached millions.

In 1972, he published **Dr. Atkins Diet Revolution**[17]. In it, he leveraged his decade of clinical experience with the low carbohydrate diet – valuable clinical experience that many of his critics had none of. Atkins asserted that one could lose weight on his diet without hunger, that blood lipids and especially triglycerides improved despite an appropriate fat intake, and that 'balanced diets' did not work because they failed to deal with the underlying disturbance in carbohydrate metabolism commonly seen in obese individuals.

This book sold half a million copies in its first 6 months, and the reaction was as dramatic as it was predictable. Harvard's Fred Stare wrote: "Any book that recommends unlimited amounts of meat, butter, and eggs, as this does, in my opinion is dangerous. The author who makes the suggestion is guilty of malpractice." Columbia's Ted Van Itallie denounced the Atkins Diet in an editorial in JAMA in 1973[18], declaring it full of "gross inaccuracies". In response, testifying before Senator McGovern's Select Committee, Dr. Atkins countered with:

"It is incredible that in 20th-century America a consci-
entious physician should have his hard-won professional
reputation placed on the line for daring to suggest that an
obesity victim might achieve some relief by cutting out
sugars and starches."

With that exchange, the battle lines were drawn, and the polemics played
out over the next three decades until Dr. Atkins' death from a head injury
caused by a fall. In that period, Dr. Atkins sold tens of millions of copies of his books, while his critics steadfastly defended the superiority of dietary carbohydrate over fat. In the meantime, serious scientists interested
in the objective evaluation of carbohydrate restricted diets found the NIH
and other granting agencies hostile to their research applications. As a result, little meaningful research was done to address the important questions
about the safety and efficacy of carbohydrate restriction, and that which
was done got shunted into obscurity. (For examples of this, see Chapter 12).

Atkins Was Not The Only One

The series of books by Dr. Robert Atkins was not the only voice in
support of low carbohydrate diets. There have been many other
books published on the topic, some bad and some good. Among the
latter, we recommend looking at the "Protein Power" books by Drs.
Michael and Mary Dan Eades[1], and also the work of Dr. Richard K.
Bernstein[2] advocating the use of carbohydrate restriction in type 1
diabetics (the latter under close medical supervision).

Senator McGovern's Dietary Guidelines

The official expression of the low fat diet hypothesis was Senator McGovern's Senate Select Committee mentioned above. Between 1976 and 1980,
this group set the agenda for who would testify and what would be decided vis-a-vis national dietary guidelines. The workings of this committee are discussed in detail in *Good Calories, Bad Calories*[13]. But it was

clear from the beginning that the outcome would be in favor of reduced dietary fat and cholesterol independent of what the science showed.

Unfortunately, this bureaucratic intransigence in the face of data has not slackened. After their initial goals and guidelines between 1977 and 1980, the results of the MRFIT and LRC studies came in and were summarily ignored. Starting from Dr. Handler's position in 1980 *"Those who argue either position strongly are expressing their values; they are not making scientific judgments"*, the MRFIT study gave a negative result and the LRC study came out statistically even. Nonetheless, the advocacy for a low fat, low cholesterol national policy lumbered forward.

Why? By the mid1980s, what had changed was that now the academic mainstream decided that there was more butter (or maybe 'low fat spread' better fits the analogy) on the 'conformity side of the bread'. No one within the academic community with Dr. Handler's courage and stature chose to stand up to question the king's wardrobe. But because the MRFIT and LRC studies had 'failed', and also because both of these large studies had failed to included women as subjects, it was decided that a new study should be done to demonstrate the benefits of a low fat, high carbohydrate diet in women.

The Women's Health Initiative (WHI)

The ultimate, and also the most expensive, test of the low fat heart disease hypothesis was the WHI launched in 1991. This massive study of 50,000 women tried to simultaneously address a number of health issues in women, including (but not limited to) the purported benefits of a low fat diet. The participants were randomized to various treatments, including a group that was aggressively counseled to reduce their dietary fat to 20% of daily energy intake (which implies a goal of at least 65% of energy from carbohydrate).

After 8 years, when the WHI investigators tallied the data, this low fat group was found to have no reduction in heart disease, stroke, breast cancer, or colon cancer compared to the group that stayed on their usual diet (about 37% fat). Simply put, a vigorously promoted low fat diet rich in complex carbohydrates, fruits and vegetables didn't seem to be all that healthful after all. Rather than admit that their carefully defended paradigm might be flawed, the study's proponents set about parsing the data to explain why their politically ordained "healthy diet" didn't work in this case.

Nor did they adequately address criticism of their protocol design that had been openly expressed from the outset of the study. Credible critics had previously noted that the WHI study design was strongly biased in favor of their low fat diet[13]. Thus the lack of a positive result is all the more surprising, implying that telling women to reduce dietary fat may have harmed their health.

The Food and Nutrition Board 2010

Now it is almost a decade after the WHI results have been tallied and digested, and we've seen many new studies published pertaining to carbohydrate-restricted diets. So we're making progress, right? Well, not if we look at the recent (June 2010) report of the US Dietary Guidelines Advisory Committee (DGAC). This group of 13 nutrition experts (appointed by the Food and Nutrition Board – the group formerly chaired by Dr. Handler, who had advised caution about the original low fat guidelines) is tasked with recommending nutrient intakes for the US population. On the topic of dietary carbohydrate intake, they advised the USDA to define the minimum human requirement for dietary carbohydrate at 130 grams per day. And in their conclusions on low carbohydrate diets, the DGAC states[19]:

> *"Diets that are less than 45% carbohydrate or more than 35% protein are difficult to adhere to, are not more effective than other calorie-controlled diets for weight loss and weight maintenance, and may pose health risk, and are therefore not recommended for weight loss or maintenance."*

In other words the DGAC report is telling ALL Americans to consume at least 45% of their calories as carbohydrate, that there is no benefit to consuming less than this amount, and that in fact it may be dangerous to do so.

Let's look at specific statements by this committee pertaining to carbohydrate.

- Carbohydrates (sugars and starches) provide energy to cells in the body, ***particularly the brain, which is a carbohydrate-dependent organ***. (italics added)

- An Estimated Average Requirement (EAR) for carbohydrate is established based on the average amount of glucose utilized by the brain.

- The Recommended Dietary Allowance (RDA) for carbohydrate is set at 130 g/d for adults and children.

What is remarkable to those of us with expertise in human metabolism is the DGAC's statement that the human brain is carbohydrate dependent, thereby mandating a high intake of dietary carbohydrate. Interestingly, this was written not by lawyers and journalists like the original McGovern Committee report, but by a committee of physicians and PhD scientists. They should know better.

In fact, the human brain is a carbohydrate-dependent organ **ONLY** if one routinely eats a lot of anti-ketogenic nutrients such as sugars and concentrated carbohydrates. When dietary carbohydrates are held to 50 grams or less per day, humans undergo a process called keto-adapation, causing the liver to make and release ketones into the bloodstream. After a few weeks of the keto-adaptation process, serum ketones increase several-fold, reaching 1-3 millimolar (mM).

Above 1 mM ketones, more than half of the brain's fuel comes from ketones. The rest of the brain's fuel must indeed come from glucose, but this amount (usually less than 50 grams per day) is easily produced endogenously by the liver from 'metabolic left-overs' via a process called gluconeogenesis. Thus, the brain uses glucose in varying amounts depending upon the availability of ketones. The manifest ability of the body to supply the brain with fuel independent of dietary carbohydrate intake clearly contradicts this committee's assertion that the brain is a carbohydrate-dependent organ. Simply put, this is a classic case of a false premise leading to a false conclusion.

The DGAC's second statement, that low carbohydrate diets "may be dangerous" was referenced to two published epidemiological studies from Europe[20, 21]. However the committee members were also likely aware of a similar study done in the United States and about to be published by Harvard researchers[22]. This recent report evaluated the reported food intakes from the Nurses Health Study and Health Professionals Follow-up Study, which looked at health outcomes over 20-26 years. Dividing the subjects into subgroups based upon reported dietary carbohydrate intakes, the Harvard researchers found a slight but statistically significant increase in mortality (~20%) in the group with the lowest intake of carbs.

Based on these data, this influential group of authors declared most low carbohydrate diets, particularly those containing animal products, as probably unsafe. Interestingly, the lowest carbohydrate intake group in the Harvard study cohort reported they consumed 37% of dietary energy as carbs, which translates into 185 grams per day for a person consuming 2000 Calories per day. Obviously this level of carbohydrate intake is well above the level of restriction shown to facilitate fat mobilization associated with nutritional ketosis.

Thus virtually no one within these study groups was keto-adapted, and this report has little relevance to the degree of carbohydrate restriction addressed in this book. As an aside, it is curious to note that this "low" level of carbohydrate intake that is deemed to be unsafe (185 grams per day) is well above the minimum intake (130 grams per day) regarded by the Dietary Guidelines Advisory Committee to be at the lower limit of safety.

However, the most powerful argument against accepting this caution about low carbohydrate diets expressed by the Harvard researchers is the fact that it was this same analytical technique, some of the same authors, and one of these two study cohorts (the Nurses Health Study) that led us down the flawed path of prescribing hormone replacement therapy (HRT) to prevent heart disease back in the 1990s. Only after the prospective, randomized Women's Health Initiative data were analyzed did we (and they) discover that HRT actually causes heart attacks (and some forms of cancer) rather than prevents them. So after it was demonstrated to yield incorrect results then, it is fascinating that these same authors now trot out the same 'dead-on-arrival' analytical method in an attempt to discredit low carbohydrate diets.

Some of the members of the Dietary Guidelines Advisory Committee know and understand these facts. So why did they cave to the consensus and put their names on the committee's flawed report? The answer is not hard to guess. First, the committee was not chosen at random from among the hundreds of qualified scientists available to serve. It was selected to include individuals known to function well on a committee – iconoclasts need not apply. Second, the committee membership includes a number of senior leaders in the field with considerable *de facto* influence over who gets papers published and grants funded – individuals whom someone a bit less senior in the field would not want to cross.

Summary

"Those who don't know history are destined to repeat it."
  – Edmund Burke (1729-1797), British Statesman and Philosopher

One might argue about whether or not we should 'repeat history' by adopting lessons learned from our hunting and herding ancestors, who practiced carbohydrate restriction for hundreds of thousands of years. However, few would argue that recent nutrition history (1970 to present), with unprecedented increases in obesity and diabetes, has been good for us. Nonetheless, there are important lessons – albeit negative ones – to be gleaned from this recent painful experience.

Up until the 1970s, we seemed to be on a path to objectively evaluate the benefits and risks of therapeutic carbohydrate restriction. Due more to politics than science, the views of Ancel Keys gained ascendency, dietary fat was deemed toxic, and carbohydrates were promoted. As the food industry built a supporting infrastructure to produce and market low fat foods, understandably the resistance to change became all that much stronger.

Against this fortress built on sand stood low carbohydrate iconoclasts like Robert Atkins, Mike and Mary Dan Eades, and Richard K. Bernstein. But now the sand under the fortress is slowly being eroded away, thanks in no small part to the incisive analysis of Gary Taubes[13, 14]. Time will tell how soon it will fall, allowing carbohydrate restriction to be fairly and objectively evaluated. When that occurs, be it in two years or ten, carbohydrate restriction may finally achieve acceptance as a therapeutic tool in western medicine.

Chapter 4

COMMON CONCERNS AT A GLANCE

We hope you feel comfortable with this historical perspective of low carbohydrate diets. However, in all likelihood you will hear strong reservations from others about adopting this lifestyle for yourself or prescribing it to your patients/clients. At this point in the book, we thought it would be helpful to briefly address common issues that people raise about carbohydrate restricted diets. These will be addressed in detail in following chapters.

1. It's Mostly Water and Muscle

Issue: Yeah, you lose pounds faster on low carb, but it's mostly water and muscle rather than body fat.

Response: The survival of this myth over the last 30 years is so amazing that we devote part of Chapter 12 (Low Carbohydrate Research Pitfalls) to a discussion of why this has occurred. In short, there is now overwhelming evidence that not only do groups of people randomized to a low carb diet lose more weight than on higher carb intakes, but they also lose more body fat. The myth of water and muscle loss came from brief studies (a few weeks or less) in people who never completed the adaptation phase of the low carb diet, in which there is often substantial water loss because of the diuretic effects of the diet. If you lose 5 pounds of fat and 5 pounds of water in the first 2 weeks, yes, half of your initial weight loss was not from fat. But if you then stay on the diet for 18 more weeks, losing two-and-a-half pounds of fat per week (but keeping all of your muscle), after 20 weeks you've lost 55 pounds, 50 of which was body fat. How to get this result, losing almost all fat and retaining or even increasing your strength and well-being, is explained as the sum of many factors which together we define as 'a well-formulated low carb diet'. To fully understand how to do this and why, you'll need to read the rest of this book.

2. Carbs are Critical

Issue: We need carbohydrate for energy, especially when we exercise.

Response: Yes, carbs do provide one source of energy for your muscles and brain, but both of these organs have completely adequate alternatives derived from dietary fat. And here's the key fact in this discussion: a high carbohydrate diet blocks your ability to employ fat to fuel your brain, and to some degree, your muscles as well. As noted in the next chapter, there is no other reason we have to include carbohydrates in the diet, which is another way of saying carbohydrates are *not* an essential dietary nutrient. However, just because carbs are not essential from a dietary perspective is not reason enough to restrict them. The real question is whether limiting carbs will adversely affect your ability to exercise. The answer is a definitive NO. When carbs are restricted to the point of inducing nutritional ketosis, the body has a remarkable capacity to transition to burning fat, even during exercise. Thirty years ago, Dr. Phinney did a study showing that fat supplied almost all of the energy used by high caliber cyclists after they had adapted to a ketogenic diet (see Chapter 10, Body Composition and Physical Performance; also Ref[23]). These guys had no problem performing high level exercise with very little dietary carbohydrate. So don't buy into the clever marketing by manufacturers promoting all those sugary sports and energy drinks. The reality is that you can exercise just fine without them when you have experienced the keto-adaption that comes after several weeks of a very low carbohydrate diet.

3.   Fear of Fat

Issue: My doctor or dietitian agrees that a low carbohydrate diet might help me lose weight, but s/he's concerned about eating too much fat long term.

Response: This is a case of good news/bad news. Your health care team appears to be supportive of a low carbohydrate diet. That's the good news. The bad news is that they still view fat as harmful under all dietary conditions. However, when you are keto-adapted, fat becomes your body's favorite fuel. But if you simultaneously restrict carbohydrate and also fat, the only other source of energy left to put on your plate is protein, and excessive consumption of protein is not a good idea. So logically fat has to be part of a properly formulated low carbohydrate diet. Particularly after you transition to weight maintenance, when your daily energy intake needs to equal your daily expenditure, consuming adequate fat becomes essential. Simply put, a key message in this book is that fat is your friend when you are on a low carbohydrate diet.

4.   Ketone Confusion

Issue: Low carbohydrate diets cannot be good for me because as a side effect my body makes toxic ketones.

Response: Very low carbohydrate diets do indeed increase production of ketones as a result of accelerated rates of fat breakdown and delivery of fatty acids to the liver. This is perfectly natural and in fact represents a rather clever and vital adaptation in fuel partitioning when your carbohydrate intake is low. When carbohydrate is restricted to less than 50 grams per day, fat breakdown is increased markedly, and blood ketones increase moderately. This state of nutritional ketosis results in ketone levels way below those characteristic of uncontrolled type-1 diabetes. This greater than 10-fold difference between nutritional ketosis and diabetic ketoacidosis (discussed in Chapter 1) is like the difference between a gentle rain and a torrential downpour. After a week or two of this moderate increase in ketone production, many of the cells in your body switch from using glucose to ketones for their primary fuel. This process of keto-adaptation is a powerful metabolic state because it means your cells have a sustained fuel supply thanks to a steady release of energy from body fat!

5. Banish the Saturated Fat Demon

Issue: Maybe an appropriate fat diet isn't necessarily bad, but I still have to avoid all those dangerous saturated fats.

Response: **IF** 'you are what you eat', and **IF** saturated fats from the diet had been proven to cause death and destruction, then this might be a valid concern. Let's take a quick look at each one in turn. We have done both human and animal studies examining the amounts of saturated fats in blood and tissue samples after a low fat, high carbohydrate diet versus a low carbohydrate diet containing appropriate fat. In both cases, the fat-containing diet provided about three times as much saturated fat. And yet, we saw no increase in saturated fat levels in either blood or tissue samples. In fact, in people with metabolic syndrome, the appropriate-fat, low carb diet actually decreased their blood levels of saturated fat, whereas the low fat diet subjects saw no decrease in blood saturates. This paradox – eating a saturate-rich diet makes your blood levels of saturates go down – occurs because keto-adapted people dramatically increase the rate that their bodies burn saturated fat. When you cut back on carbo-hydrates to the point that fats get burned first, the saturated fats go to the front of the line, and if you burn them up for energy before they can ac-cumulate, how are they going to harm you?

In response to the second 'IF', scientists have begun to take a second look at the 50-year old idea that dietary saturated fats are harmful. Yes, it has been shown that saturated fats in animal or human diets can raise blood cholesterol under some circumstances. However, we now know that some forms of blood cholesterol are either not harmful or even protective (like HDL cholesterol), and a well-formulated low carb diet containing a fair amount of saturated fat has been shown repeatedly to raise blood levels of this 'good cholesterol'. Moreover, three studies published in the last year have examined carefully collected dietary records of huge populations who were followed for decades. In all of three of these recent studies, there was no connection between saturated fat intake and either the frequency of heart attack or death[24-26].

If it doesn't accumulate when you eat it, and eating it hasn't been shown to actually harm you, where's the demon in saturated fat?

6. Feeling Faint

Issue: I'm happy losing weight with a low carbohydrate diet, but I'm always tired, get light headed when I stand up, and if I exercise for more than 10 minutes I feel like I'm going to pass out.

Response: Congratulations on your weight loss success, and with just a small adjustment to your diet, you can say goodbye to your weakness and fatigue. The solution is salt…a bit **more** salt to be specific. This may sound like we're crazy when many experts argue that we should all eat less salt, however these are the same experts who tell us that eating lots of carbohydrates and sugar is OK. But what they don't tell you is that your body functions very differently when you are keto-adapted. When you restrict carbs for a week or two, your kidneys switch from retaining salt to rapidly excreting it, along with a fair amount of stored water. This salt and water loss explains why many people experience rapid weight loss in the first couple of weeks on a low carbohydrate diet.

Ridding your body of this excess salt and water is a good thing, but only up to a point. After that, if you don't replace some of the ongoing sodium excretion, the associated water loss can compromise your circulation The end result is lightheadedness when you stand up quickly or fatigue if you exercise enough to get 'warmed up'. Other common side effects of carbohydrate restriction that go away with a pinch of added salt include headache and constipation; and over the long term it also helps the body maintain its muscles. The best solution is to include 1 or 2 cups of bouillon or broth in your daily schedule. This adds only 1-2 grams of sodium to your daily intake, and your keto-adapted metabolism insures that you pass it right on through within a matter of hours (allaying any fears you might have of salt buildup in your system).

This rapid clearance also means that on days that you exercise, take one dose of broth or bouillon within the hour before you start.

7. Short vs Sustained Weight Loss

Issue: I am ready to try a low carbohydrate diet for weight loss, but once I've reached my goal my dietitian tells me I need to switch to a diet with lots of whole grains and other healthy carbohydrates.

Response: Unfortunately, all too frequently people lose weight on a low carbohydrate diet and then promptly regain it all back. Why? A common reason is they failed to view a low carbohydrate diet as a lifestyle. If you respond really well to a low carbohydrate diet as a weight loss tool, part of the reason is your willpower, but the other reason is that your body is probably not good at processing carbohydrates. For most people, this difficulty metabolizing carbohydrates does not go away even after you've lost some weight. So after losing 15 or 150 pounds, if you transition back to a diet with too much carbohydrate, you will likely regain much of the weight, even if the carbs you eat are the apparent 'healthy' ones. Yes, it is possible that you might be able to add some carbs back into your diet once you have reached your goal weight, but be very cautious. Listen to your body as much if not more than you listen to your dietitian. Adding back too much carbohydrate can put you on a slippery slope back to your former weight. To prepare yourself for long term success, from the very start you need to view your low carbohydrate diet as a permanent lifestyle, not just a temporary weight loss tool.

8. Moderation Madness

Issue: Restricting an entire macronutrient class seems extreme – especially carbohydrates which are known to give us quick energy. We should be encouraging moderation in all foods and a balanced diet.

Response: This is one of the more common comments we hear. After all, how can you argue against quick energy, moderation and balance? The answer depends to some degree on preconceptions around the meaning of moderation and what you consider 'good' nutrition. If consuming lots of carbohydrate provided some essential nutrient that would otherwise be lacking, then we might agree that a low carbohydrate diet is unbalanced or even extreme. But that's clearly not the case. Think of it this way – what if you lived in California and planned a vacation in Hawaii. Would you believe someone who told you going that far was 'extreme', and therefore you ought to try flying just half way there instead? In this analogy, practicing this form of moderation would land you in seriously deep water. 'Moderation' and 'balanced' are meaningless terms when we are talking about 'islands of safety'. And if your body is carbohydrate intolerant, eating a low carbohydrate diet is your island of dietary safety. Should a person with gluten intolerance consume moderate amounts of gluten so they can have a balanced diet? Of course not. Then why should a person with carbohydrate intolerance consume moderate amounts of carbs to meet some arbitrary criterion of a 'balanced' diet? From the point of view of essential nutrients and adequate energy to power your body, a low carbohydrate diet is 'balanced'. Yes, this does mean that carbohydrates as a non-essential nutrient class are restricted, but you can still get all of the essential nutrients and energy your body needs by selecting from a broad array of natural low carbohydrate foods.

9. Missing Micronutrients

Issue: You can't get all the vitamins and minerals you need for health on a low carbohydrate diet.

Response: If you choose from a variety of naturally low carbohydrate foods (e.g., eggs, fish, meats, poultry, nuts, seeds, berries, cheese, olive and canola oils, cream, butter, and a vast array of vegetables) you'll automatically achieve adequate intake of all the essential vitamins and minerals. But where do you get your vitamin C if you can't drink orange juice? How about Brussels sprouts, peppers, cauliflower, kale, and broccoli? All are excellent sources of vitamin C. Also, half a cup of berries per day can provide quite a bit of vitamin C. For example, there's 42 mg of vitamin C – half of the daily recommended intake – (and only 5 grams of carbs) in half a cup of fresh strawberries.

10. Brittle Bones and Kidney Crisis

Issue: I have heard that diets like Atkins which are low in carbohydrate and high in protein may cause my bones to weaken and my kidneys to fail.

Response: First of all, a well-formulated low carbohydrate diet like Atkins is not really that high in protein. We recommend protein between 1.5 and 2.0 grams per kilogram reference body weight (0.7 to 0.9 grams per pound reference weight). This translates to between 90 and 150 grams per day for a range of adults, which is about what the average adult in the US is already eating. This level is well tolerated and is not associated with adverse effects on bone, kidney or other health indictors. The reason that protein intakes higher than the minimum recommended (0.8 grams per kilogram) were thought to negatively impact bone is because they cause a small but measureable increase in urinary calcium excretion. On the surface, this could indicate a higher risk for bone loss over time and development of osteoporosis. However, we now know that increasing dietary protein above the minimum also causes greater intestinal absorption of dietary calcium, which balances the slightly greater calcium loss in the urine. In fact, recent research suggests that diets higher in protein are associated with healthier bones as people age.

Similar to the situation with bone health, the concern about kidney problems stems from a belief that high protein diets contribute to renal disease. This belief is based on studies of restricting protein in people who already have severely damaged kidneys. However, there is no data linking the moderate protein intake range listed above to damage in people with normal kidney function. In technical terms, despite some evidence that higher protein intakes can increase glomerular filtration rate, the evidence linking this normal physiologic response to progressive loss of kidney function in healthy people is completely lacking.

Chapter 5

DIETARY CARBOHYDRATES: SCIENTIFIC AND CULTURAL PERSPECTIVES

Introduction

As the previous chapter indicates, we are used to responding to the litany of concerns that are raised about low carbohydrate diets. Typically, our responses to these questions involve a short answer and a published reference or two. (Well, maybe some of Steve Phinney's answers are a bit more extensive…) The typical result of these interactions is that people are surprised and impressed by the quality of science supporting low carbohydrate nutrition.

However, one particularly stubborn issue that still troubles a good number of people can be encapsulated as a fundamental belief that *very low carbohydrate diets are not balanced*. And few would argue that an unbalanced diet is healthy. In essence, this is a case where a diet is sabotaged simply by how its critics frame it conceptually. No matter that our response might have an excellent basis of scientific support, if we let the low carb diet be framed as 'unbalanced', it's game over.

How do we respond to professional colleagues and family/friends who have such a mind-set? While this issue was addressed briefly as 'Point 8' in the preceding chapter, it is complex enough that we feel the need to devote this chapter to addressing it more fully. There are a couple of important points that deserve careful discussion, and these are relevant to your decision whether or not to remain on the fence about the safety and efficacy of low carbohydrate diets.

Defining a Balanced Diet

We like to promote moderation and a balanced lifestyle for many good reasons. We can all agree that balancing competing factors like work demands with quality family time, or physical exercise with relaxation, is desirable. But when we carry that over to diet, 'balance' is too often arbitrarily translated into eating relatively equal proportions of macronutrients from a variety of foods.

Whereas this may work for many people, we have tried to make the case in this book that a subset of people (particularly those with insulin resistance) manifest themselves as having varying degrees of carbohydrate intolerance. Within this subgroup, some may remain healthy and functional by consuming 100 grams per day of carbohydrate, whereas others need to restrict this macronutrient down to 30 or 40 grams per day to avoid overt diabetes, obesity, or hypertension. So should the same 'balanced diet' in respect to carbohydrate, protein and fat be recommended to these individuals as the rest of the general population?

Unfortunately, that judgment may depend on one's preconceived notion of a 'balanced diet'. We don't bat a therapeutic eyelash when we restrict gluten if a person has Celiac disease, or restrict lactose (milk sugar) in a person with lactose intolerance. Also consider the perspective of our pre-agricultural ancestors who consumed relatively little carbohydrate for hundreds of thousands of years before modern agriculture practices became dominant. And even into relatively modern times, the highly evolved hunting cultures of the Inuit and North American Bison People or the herding culture of the Masai offer testimony to the ability of humans to thrive in the virtual absence of concentrated dietary carbohydrates.

From the perspective of an Inuit or Lakota grandmother, our current agri-business diet would appear to be anything but 'balanced'. Balance is a relative term, and its antithesis, 'unbalanced', is clearly defined by one's cultural baseline. So let's try to take off our cultural blinders and look at the sources of this concept that a substantial percentage of carbohydrate (be it 30% or 60%) is an obligate component of a 'balanced diet'.

Carbohydrate as an Essential Nutrient Class

A root concept of dietary need is 'essentiality'. If no single component within a macronutrient class is essential to human well-being or function, then it is hard to argue in favor of a need for that macronutrient. And if we take that macronutrient away from the diets of individuals or whole cultures and they continue to thrive for a year or for millennia, case closed. Agreed?

In the last century, nutrition science defined nine amino acids (leucine, isoleucine, valine, threonine, tryptophan, phenylalanine, tyrosine, histidine, and maybe cysteine) as essential. Specifically, that means that they must be supplied by the diet because they cannot be produced by the body in adequate amounts to meet metabolic need for protein synthesis. Without these essential amino acids over a matter of weeks or months, protein metabolism is impaired and disease and dysfunction ensue.

Similarly, between 1929 and 1978, two essential fatty acid families (the omega-6 and omega-3 classes) were defined. If these polyunsaturated fats are not sufficient in the diet over months (omega-6) or over decades (omega-3), then overt disease and dysfunction occur. Omega-6 deficiency causes skin rash, growth stunting and sterility. Omega-3 deficiency causes heart disease (and possibly dementia) in the first generation, plus impaired neurological/visual/intellectual development in the second generation.

But where is the evidence for essentiality for any single molecule or structural class within dietary carbohydrates. What are the signs and symptoms characteristic of carbohydrate deficiency? Fatigue? No, not if a modicum of sodium and a modest period of adaptation are allowed. Growth impairment? No, the pre-contact Osage, and Kiowa in North America and the Masai in Africa were giants by modern standards. Impaired intellectual development? Well, the people of the Pacific Northwest were living in large wooden houses and processing and storing oolichan grease millennia before the development of olive oil in the Eastern Mediterranean.

So what are the textbook characteristics of dietary carbohydrate deficiency? Yes, we agree that maintaining a normal blood glucose level is essential for human well-being. But the key question is: how is that linked to dietary carbohydrate intake? The spoilers here for those claiming the essentiality of dietary carbs are the terms 'gluconeogenesis' and 'adaptation', which allow us to maintain normal blood glucose levels without dietary carbohydrate.

Gluconeogenesis is the combination of pathways through which our metabolism collects and revises the carbon skeletons of amino acids, the glycerol backbones from triglycerides, and even lactic acid to make new glucose to feed those few tissues (like the lens of the eye and red blood cells) that can't burn either fat or ketones.

Adaptation is the process through which whole organs in the body forgo glucose (from muscle to brain) and switch to burning mostly fat for fuel. The combination of gluconeogenesis and adaptation together is what allowed a group of bike racers studied by Steve Phinney to eat no visible carbohydrate for 4 weeks and still show up and perform well in their second exercise test[23]. But in light of Stefansson's do-or-die performance in the 1928 Bellevue Study (Chapter 2), this was no big surprise.

So what does this mean? It means that we should not confuse our body's ability to maintain a normal blood glucose with our dietary carbohydrate intake. When humans are adapted to a low carbohydrate diet, blood sugar levels and one's carbohydrate intake are completely independent of one another. In fact, keto-adapted humans maintain better glucose levels across feeding, fasting, and extremes of exercise than when fed a low fat, high carbohydrate diet[23, 27].

How about sports performance? Don't athletes perform better when given a high carbohydrate diet? That was the accepted paradigm 20-30 years ago, but it has not stood the test of time for many endurance sports.

48

Even some weight lifters and other strength/power athletes are now training and performing on carbohydrate restricted diets. This works to their benefit in part because of an ability to maintain a lower body fat content without losing muscle size and function and also an improved perception of 'recovery' between workouts. But here is the key question. Even if someone can run a mile a bit faster on a high carbohydrate diet than on one restricted in carbohydrates, is this evidence for dietary essentiality? If that were true, then both caffeine and ephedra (both of which improve performance) could also be classed as essential nutrients.

Carbohydrate as a Cultural (if not Religious) Imperative

Christianity arose in a region where wheat was the staff of life. Every Christian recognizes the phrase "give us this day, our daily bread". This very quickly becomes thin ice for a scientist when there is no emotional daylight between dietary carbohydrate and our instinctive (or religious) sense of well-being, and thus our very existence. It is a religious tenet and thus defies being questioned.

The point here is that there is a very blurry line between our rational and emotional attraction to dietary carbohydrates. Specifically, do we as scientists rationally examine the possibility that our intellectual constructs of dietary essentiality shadow our religious beliefs? Perhaps rarely. Does it affect our thinking and actions? Almost certainly.

But is this zeal to promote dietary carbohydrate purely a function of Christianity or religion in general? Obviously not. As agriculture became a dominant force around the globe, the majority of those early farmers were not yet able to read or count. That left the decision of when to sow and when to harvest in the hands of the learned class in any society, be they chiefs, priests or shamans. This empowered a leadership class in most agrarian societies, and they appropriately recognized that the origin of their power emanated from agricultural carbohydrates.

Now fast forward to the present in North America. Who rules our thinking about dietary principles? Is it the academic nutrition community (aka, scientists)? Doctors? Dietitians? Agri-business? The US Department of Agriculture? Oprah? We don't have a definitive answer to this question. But if we look objectively at where the money and power lie, there is little doubt that culture, religion, industry, and government are complicit in the subjective decision to discount the science supporting low carbohydrate diets.

When we think about it in this light, the 'Hail Mary' tactic of claiming that low carbohydrate diets are imbalanced is linguistically spot on!

Low Carbohydrate Diets are Extreme

The belief that a low carbohydrate diet is unbalanced is often expressed another way – it's labeled 'extreme'. Because it is viewed as extreme in the restriction of a macronutrient we happen to cherish as a cultural icon, there is an analogous perception that the diet is unpalatable and difficult to adhere to over time. In fact, many believe the main reason for weight loss success with carbohydrate restriction is because of the monotony of the diet. The views that consuming a low carbohydrate diet takes Spartan-like discipline, or that food choices are severely limited, are some of the most commonly claimed deterrents to their use.

That a low carbohydrate diet must be draconian, lacking both palatability and the ability to elicit pleasure could not be further from the truth. The actual experience of most people who choose to follow a well-formulated low carbohydrate diet is that it is highly satisfying. In fact, the ease with which one's hunger is satisfied while eating copious amounts of vegetables and delicious fat-containing foods (knowing that this fat flows directly to cells for energy rather than storage) sound pretty empowering – and that's how many people describe it.

And for those who happen to have even a small degree of culinary curiosity, there are almost infinite combinations of naturally low carbohydrate ingredients that can be incorporated into delectable meals. So far from being simply bacon and eggs at every meal, the ability to experiment with a wide variety of ingredients can be an incredibly enjoyable aspect to the low carbohydrate experience (see sidebar).

Consider this menu for a dinner the authors shared while writing this book

New York strip steak grilled with an Italian herb rub

Mushrooms sautéed in olive oil and garlic

Garden-fresh green beans, steamed and buttered

Caprese salad (heirloom tomato, fresh mozzarella, basil leaves, and a honey-basil-roasted garlic vinaigrette)

Home-made maple walnut ice cream

Total carbohydrate for the meal: 25 grams. Total Calories: 1000-1200

(see Chapter 17 for more examples of the succulent variety in the authors' diets)

Summary

What should you think when you hear consensus experts discount low carbohydrate diets as 'unbalanced'? What should you think when doctors or dietitians state that humans need to eat a lot of carbohydrates? Please don't think 'conspiracy'. We firmly believe that our colleagues don't secretly meet and decide how they are going to present a united front against a low carbohydrate diet insurgency. We doubt they even think of us as insurgent. They just think of us as 'wrong', where 'wrong' is based more on their cultural and religious identity than on science.

These are powerful forces that shape what we think and what we are willing to question. But both history and modern science tell us that, rather than being physiologically required for normal metabolism, dietary carbohydrates are an optional macronutrient for humans. Blood sugar levels are well maintained in the keto-adapted individual, even across intense exercise. There is no textbook entity or clinical condition characteristic of dietary carbohydrate deficiency.

As you read on in this book, you might come to view the decision to eat a low or high carbohydrate diet as a simple trade-off. If you have underlying insulin resistance, do you want to eat carbs and struggle unsuccessfully with your weight, or forego them and be thinner? If you have type-2 diabetes, do you want to have a "balanced diet" or do you want to come off your pills and insulin while putting your diabetes into remission by adopting a well-formulated low carbohydrate diet? For many people, these benefits make it worth the effort to set aside a cultural dietary icon in favor of better health and well-being.

Section 3

PHYSIOLOGY

Chapter 6

BASIC HUMAN ENERGETICS AND FUEL PARTITIONING

Introduction

To appreciate how human energy metabolism adapts when dietary carbo-hydrates are reduced, it helps to have a basic understanding of what fuels we burn and where we burn them. This topic is labeled 'fuel partitioning' because different cells and different organs in our bodies use and store different fuels. The focus here is not on biochemistry (i.e., enzymes and pathways), but on the physiology of human fuel use – how the body's organs acquire the fuel they need to function from either food or from stored energy reserves.

For this purpose, you need to know a bit about energy units (see side-bar), and the tools we use to assess human energy use. The advanced reader may be tempted to skim through this chapter, as it provides basic information to allow a range of readers to fully appreciate the complexity and adaptability of human energy metabolism. However, the concept of keto-adaptation, the key to understanding fuel partitioning during carbo-hydrate restriction, is explained herein and is best not neglected.

"Calories"

When we use the term "calorie" in reference to human energetics, we really mean a "Calorie", which is the same as a kilocalorie. In correct use, a "calorie" with a lower case "c" is the amount of energy needed to raise 1 cc of water by one degree Centigrade. Thus a kilocalorie (kcal) will raise a <u>liter</u> of water by 1° C.

<u>Clinical Example</u>. So how does this apply to human energetics? This makes sense when you think about the common practice of "warming up" when exercising. A lean person's body contains between 50 and 80 kg of "stuff" (i.e., 50-80 liters, most of which is water, see Body Composition, below) that needs to be heated up. So if you start exercising at a rate that expends say 400 Calories per hour, you will have burned about 100 Calories in 15 minutes. Since most of the fuel we burn ends up as heat, that means in 15 minutes you would have generated enough heat to bring your temperature up between 1-2°C – from normal 37°C to about 38.5°C. Thus, at that point in an exercise session, you are "warmed up" – literally. After that, since 38.5 °C is the human fever threshold, any additional heat generated by exercise must be dissipated by radiation, convection, or evaporation of sweat to avoid developing a high fever, heat prostration, or heat stroke.

Carbohydrate Metabolism

Most carbohydrates provide about 4 Calories per gram in their pure dry form. However, most prepared carbohydrate foods (fresh bread, cooked rice/pasta/potato, juices) contain more water than carbohydrate, which "dilutes" out the calorie count somewhat. Thus 100 grams of mashed potatoes contains only 100 Calories or so (before you add the butter or gravy!). Granulated sugar, on the other hand, is pure dry carbohydrate, so the 4 grams in a level teaspoon provides 16 Calories. Once eaten, most carbohydrates are digested and turned into glucose, which is also what we commonly call blood sugar. The one major exception to this rule is fructose, which metabolically cannot be made directly into glucose (see sidebar).

Fructose – a sugar that partitions like fat

Most of the fructose we eat, whether as sucrose (table sugar), high fructose corn sweetener, or in natural fruits and fruit juice gets made into fat by our liver. This is because our body can't convert fructose to glucose, and the first step in cellular fructose metabolism diverts it away from the primary pathway of glucose metabolism (the Myerhoff-Embden pathway). Thus these two 6-carbon sugars, fructose and glucose, follow separate metabolic paths. In the case of fructose, it is cleaved into two 3-carbon fragments, both of which primarily contribute to fat production (lipogenesis) in the liver.

Twisted Logic? Most energy drinks and sports beverages use sucrose or high fructose corn sweetener as their primary energy source. Given that the average exhausted athlete still has tens of thousands of fat calories in body energy reserves but is running out of carbohydrate (glycogen), why would one want to add a sugar that cannot be used for quick energy, with most of it eventually ending up as fat?

At any point in time in a healthy non-diabetic individual, there are just a couple of "teaspoons" of free glucose (about 40 Calories worth) in the body's circulation (i.e., the bloodstream). This means that when you digest and absorb a cup of mashed potatoes or rice, most of the 200 Calories of glucose entering the bloodstream when it gets digested has to be rapidly cleared to someplace else to keep blood sugar in the normal range. If it weren't, blood sugar would rise to more than twice normal within 2 hrs after a meal, and you'd have an instant case of diabetes. Both types of diabetes are diseases caused by the body's inability to dispose of glucose entering the bloodstream. It comes in two general varieties – type-1 if your body can't make insulin, and type-2 if you can make insulin but your cells tend to ignore the insulin signal (aka insulin resistance). These diseases and their response to carbohydrate restriction are discussed in Chapter 15.

So where does glucose go when it leaves the bloodstream? Normally much of it gets taken up into muscle and burned immediately or stored as little starch-like granules (glycogen) in the cells for later use. Your liver also stores some glucose as glycogen, which it then releases to keep blood sugar normal over-night or during prolonged exercise. And some ingested glucose is used "real-time" by your brain to keep the lights on. But an adult at rest burns at most 50 kcal of glucose per hour, so at least half of that cup of mashed potatoes has to be promptly tucked away in storage, preferably as glycogen.

If you have insulin resistance, your rate of glycogen synthesis in response to eating carbohydrates is considerably impaired. Even if you're adept at storing carbs, there's only so much glycogen that your muscles and liver can store – somewhere between 1000 and 2000 Calories in an adult, depend-ing on how big your muscles are and your training status (exercise training can increase the amount of stored glycogen). So what happens when you eat more carbs than you can burn right away and your glycogen reserves are already full? Rather than let your blood sugar skyrocket up to diabetic levels, your liver, and to some degree your fat cells, go to work turning that extra glucose into fat – a process called lipogenesis. Once that glucose (or fructose) is made into fat, there is no way back – humans can't make fat back into blood sugar – so lipogenesis is a metabolic one-way street, ending in what for many people becomes a crowded parking lot (your fat cells).

Protein Metabolism

Protein consists of long chains made of 20 different amino acids that the body uses to build and maintain structures like tendons, ligaments, bone, skin, hair and nails, plus organs like muscles, kidneys, liver, intestine, and lungs. Amino acids are also used to make enzymes and membrane-bound receptors and transporters that move specific molecules (like glucose) in and out of cells. And some hormones are proteins – insulin, for example, is a 51-amino acid protein chain that stimulates glucose uptake by muscle and fat, without which that cup of mashed potatoes would be acutely toxic.

All of the body's proteins, whether in blood, muscle, brain, or bone, are in a continuous state of turnover. This is because protein containing tissues are constantly being repaired or renewed, so your body needs a consistent source of protein to maintain itself. If you don't get enough protein for a day, a week or a month, your body will allow net breakdown of some tissues in order to recycle the amino acids it needs to keep vital structures up to par. And if you are growing taller or building muscle, this further increases your   need somewhat above the minimum protein intake required for maintenance.

Current guidelines recommend 0.8 grams/day of protein per kilogram of body weight for adults, with more for children, adolescents, and pregnant women. Most people in the US get much more than this unless they are vegan or vegetarians or make really lousy food choices. So beyond this minimum, the key questions about protein are: 1) is the minimum recommended intake optimum; if not, how much is? And 2) how much is too much?

The question of defining an optimum protein dose does not have a simple answer. In addition to growth in childhood and pregnancy, multiple factors significantly alter your daily protein need. Important variables that increase an individual's protein need include energy restriction (i.e., weight loss dieting), inflammation or illness, and recovery of lean tissue after a period of loss (such as following starvation, famine, or prolonged illness).

Another factor known to influences our body's need for protein is the mix of carbohydrate and fat that provides most of the energy in our diet. However, the magnitude of this factor is very dependent on timing. In short term studies, taking away dietary carbohydrate and replacing it with fat reduces our body's efficiency in using protein. Put another way, when you first take away dietary carbs, you need more protein to maintain muscle and other protein-containing tissues. But when you observe a human over a number of weeks of adaptation to a low carbohydrate diet, most of this initial inefficiency in protein use goes away[27]. Thus, once you are keto-adapted, your body's need for protein isn't much higher than during a 'balanced diet'. This is a key fact in our understanding that low carbohydrate diets used in the long term do not need to be particularly high in protein.

All the protein we eat (with the exception of stuff that is rubbed or cut off, like skin, hair, and nails) eventually gets burned for energy, yielding 4 Calories per gram. And you can't "push" your body to build muscle by eating extra protein – muscle is built up under the stimulus of exercise (or illicit pharmaceuticals) as long as adequate protein is available at the time. No one has ever shown that more than 1.5 gram/kg improves human protein synthesis (which translates to ~100 gram/day for a 5'10" male, about what the average US omnivore eats daily (100 gram = 400 kcal = 15% of 2700 kcal). That said, however, generations of power athletes have made the empiric observation that they train and compete better on proportionately higher protein intakes (e.g., 1.5 to 2.5 grams per kg).

As for how much is too much protein, this again has not been precisely defined. As a general rule, in the short term, people start to feel "unwell" if they routinely eat more than 30% of their daily energy need as protein. Even though low carbohydrate diets are often casually identified as high protein, the truth is most may not actually be that high. One factor driving this misunderstanding is that "protein foods" like bacon, eggs, fried chicken, tuna salad, hamburger, and even lean steak typically contain more fat calories than protein calories. So in fact, "high protein" diets consisting of common foods tend to be higher in fat than protein.

Second, when someone goes on the Atkins or another low carbohydrate diet, they usually lose weight, right? Much of that weight loss comes from body fat, which typically provides the body up to half its daily energy from "inside" (i.e., endogenous stores) during the initial weight loss phase. So if someone is eating 1400 kcal/day consisting of relatively lean "protein foods" that are half protein (700 kcal) but burns 2800 kcal per day, his/her dietary protein intake is actually supplying only 25% of their total daily energy need, falling well below the empiric 30% ceiling noted above. But to the casual observer who is ignoring the contribution of body fat stores, the actual food being consumed appears to be high in protein

The other important implication of this is that when a person makes the transition from weight loss to weight maintenance on a low carbohydrate diet, total energy intake must increase. Carbohydrate necessarily remains a small fraction of one's dietary energy supply in order to remain in a keto-adapted state and avoid the side effects of carbohydrate intolerance. Therefore, the proportion of fat to protein in the diet needs to be increased to avoid overeating protein. This important issue will be discussed in more detail in Chapter 16.

Protein and Kidney Function – Lessons from Kidney Donors

In the past 50 years, tens of thousands of individuals with two healthy kidneys have donated one of them to save another's life. As a result, there are currently about 100,000 people in the US with only one kidney, with some of them surviving this way since the 1970s. None of these people are advised to eat less protein, even though they have only half as much kidney function. What this effectively does is double their protein intake relative to kidney function. Yes, the remaining kidney does get a bit bigger, but it doesn't come close to doubling in size.

Recently, within this population, only 65 have developed kidney failure and needed a transplant of their own over an approximately 3-year period. This is about half the average rate of kidney failure in the general population. And here's the kicker – most of these people gave a kidney to a relative who needed one, and the most common causes of kidney failure run in families. Based on that, we'd expect the donors to have more cases of kidney failure than the general population. This is a head-scratcher, but clearly this indicates that dietary protein is not a big killer of kidneys.

That said, dietary protein restriction is a recognized factor in preserving residual glomerular function in individuals with advanced kidney failure, but the value of extremely low protein diets in this situation remains a topic of ongoing debate. However, the extrapolation of this extreme clinical example to the presumption that dietary protein in the ranges discussed above is a primary cause of renal disease is completely unfounded.

Energy in Foods – Fat

Most fats we get from foods are triglycerides, consisting of a glycerol "backbone" with 3 fatty acid molecules attached. An additional class of dietary fat, coming from the membranes of plants and animal, is phospholipids, which tend to be higher in essential fatty acids. Both triglycerides and phospholipids can be metabolized (burned) for energy, and they provide about 9 Calories per gram.   And because many dietary fats and oils contain little or no water, fatty foods tend to be pretty energy dense (e.g., a cup of butter, olive oil, or lard contains 1600-1800 kcal).

Because fats do not dissolve in water, they are carried in the bloodstream as triglyceride droplets surrounded by emulsifying molecules like phospholipids, cholesterol, and proteins. These particles are called lipoproteins, and they are subject to much loathing because they contain cholesterol. In reality, these lipoproteins are like trucks loaded with energy traveling about in the bloodstream delivering fuel to cells. All lipoproteins contain cholesterol, and their cholesterol contents may be labeled "bad" or "good" depending on where these lipoproteins are formed and where they tend to end up. It is a simple but underappreciated fact that without cholesterol, there could be no lipoproteins, and we'd be hard pressed for an alternative method to distribute fats and fat soluble nutrients to our cells for structure and energy.

At any one point in time in a healthy person, there is more energy as fat in the circulation than as glucose, and its exchange in and out of storage in fat cells and in the liver is every bit as dynamic and important as is glucose. In another similarity to glucose, fat is also taken up by muscles for both immediate use as well as for storage. Fat storage droplets in muscle serve as reserve fuel to support exercise (just like glycogen), dropping to low levels after prolonged exercise and building back up over the next day or two of recovery.

In addition to their role as the body's primary fuel source when insulin levels are restrained, dietary fats also contain two 'families' of essential fatty acids. Identified by their uniquely positioned double (unsaturated) bonds called omega-3 and omega-6, these two classes of fatty acids serve a wide variety of structural and signaling functions throughout the body. And because their unique structures cannot be created by human metabolism, these two classes of essential fats must be consumed from dietary sources. The metabolism of these essential fatty acids is profoundly changed in the context of carbohydrate restriction, and the implications of this for intake guidelines will be discussed in Chapter 9.

Body Composition and Energy Content

People obviously vary tremendously in height and weight. However, not so obvious is the fact that two individuals of the same height and weight can vary a great deal in "body composition". Because we humans can only store a small amount of carbohydrate as glycogen (a maximum of 500 grams in a well-trained, muscular male, which is 0.6% of an 80 kg body), the biggest variations in body composition between individuals are in the relative proportions of lean tissue and fat.

Healthy normal men can have up to 20% body fat, whereas this upper limit for women is 28%. The lower limits for healthful percent body fat are less clear, in part because getting to a very low value by starvation as opposed to exercise might significantly affect one's well-being. That said, it is not unusual to find highly trained males with less than 10% body fat (and similarly under 15% in female athletes). Therefore it is possible to have two 5'10" guys weighing 170 pounds, one with 17 pounds of body fat and the other with 34 pounds, with both qualifying as normal.

The other variable with body fat is where it is located. Fat carried "centrally" (i.e., around the middle, and particularly within the abdominal cavity) is associated with greater risk for developing diabetes and heart disease than fat carried below the waist. Therefore, risk calculations based just on height and weight, and even those that attempt to measure total body fat, provide less than optimum information for an individual concerned about her/his health. In this context, a simple waist circumference sometimes offers better information on health risk than a total body fat determination by a space-age instrument.

The importance of where one carries body fat is interesting from an evolutionary perspective because the apparent role of body fat is to tide us through lean times, like famine or seasonal food shortage. When you look at pictures of people who have experienced a famine, neither bellies nor butts are preserved, which means both get mobilized when the body needs fuel. But barring total starvation, a diet or treatment that favors the loss of abdominal fat would be desirable.

Which brings us to the question: how much energy reserve does a healthy person carry, and how long will it last if there's no food? So let's take a hypothetical 5'6", 132 pound (60 kg) woman with 25% body fat set adrift in a life-boat with plenty of water and no food. Her 15 kg of adipose tissue is about 85% by weight triglyceride, so she has about 115,000 Calories of fat reserves. She can also burn about half of her body protein content (10,000 kcal of her 20,000 total) before she dies. Sitting quietly in the boat (i.e., not rowing) she'll start out burning about 2000 Calories per day. This implies that she'd last about 62 days.

But not so fast – a bunch of other things happen when a human stops eating. Remember that protein is constantly turning over throughout the body, and if there's no replacement dietary protein coming in, lean tissue is broken down and lost. The bad news is that our hypothetical subject in the boat gets weaker, but there are 2 pieces of good news. First, over a week or two, the body adapts to get by with less protein breakdown (i.e., keto-adaptation), so the rate of loss of lean tissue (i.e., muscle) slows as the weeks go by.

Second, our resting metabolism can adjust itself in response to starvation, going down 10-15% in the first few weeks, and then going down further as more and more muscle is lost. Net/net: our hardy hypothetical heroine will last somewhere between 75 and 90 days in her lifeboat. The bad news for guys is that because we typically start with about the same or less amount of body fat and more muscle (translation, higher resting metabolism), our down-hill slope is steeper and the little "X" at the end of the curve typically comes at about 60 days. Newton might have said something like "For every advantage, there's a disadvantage." Take-home message: whether you're a guy or a gal, take some food with you in the life-boat if you're a long way from land.

What Your Organs Burn

Here's a question for you – do all cells and organs in your body use the same fuels? Specifically; if your diet consists of 20% protein, 30% fat, and 50% carbs, do all cells throughout the body use this identical fuel mix? The answer, of course, is "no" (because if it were "yes", why would we be asking this question?)

Some cells prefer fats for fuel, others prefer glucose, and some are so specialized that they prefer just one particular amino acid. So no matter what you eat, it seems that some types of cells would feel deprived unless the body had a way to divvy up energy sources among organs and cells and also had alternatives when necessary. As a result, the inter-organ exchange of fuel is both complex and dynamic. Here are a few simple tastes of the complexity and elegance of this system.

Muscle: When we say muscle, we typically mean the things that move our arms and legs, technically called skeletal muscles (which differ in form and function from the cardiac muscle in our heart and also from the third type of muscle (smooth) that lines blood vessels and our gastrointestinal tract). At rest, skeletal muscles prefer fat for fuel, using glucose only when insulin levels are high and blood sugar needs some place to go. During sustained exercise, fat is still the preferred fuel at intensities up to 50-60% of that muscle's maximum continuous effort. Above 60% of maximum effort, glucose (or stored glycogen) progressively assumes a dominant role, although this dominance is attenuated when individuals are given a few weeks to adapt to a low carbohydrate diet[23, 27]. Also at these higher intensities, some of this glucose is not completely metabolized but is partially broken down to lactate and released back into the bloodstream rather than being oxidized in muscle mitochondria all the way to CO_2 and water. By contrast, during resistance exercise (very high intensity, brief duration), most of the fuel use consists of glucose made into lactate.

But here's the interesting part. Lactate has a bad reputation as a cause of muscle fatigue and pain. This is a classic case of guilt by association. During transition from rest to intense exercise, the increased production of lactic acid rapidly disassociates into lactate and hydrogen ion. It is the accumulation of hydrogen ion, not lactate per se, that contributes to fatigue due to acidosis. Lactate has a much more interesting and positive role to play in the human body. Much of the lactate released from muscle during exercise gets taken up by the liver and made back into glucose (a process called gluconeogenesis) and sent back to the muscles where it can be made into lactate again. And because the liver uses mostly fat to power gluconeogenesis, this shuttle of glucose out from the liver and lactate back (called the Cori cycle) actually ends up powering resistance exercise from energy released by fat oxidation in the liver.

Heart: The predominant fuel preferred by your heart when you are not exercising is fat. The heart rarely uses much glucose, with the only exception being during a heart attack when a vessel is plugged and the oxygen supply to that part of the muscle is cut off or severely reduced. In that case, the small amount of glycogen in heart muscle is used anaerobically to make lactate. And here's one more bit of heresy about lactate. During exercise, a healthy and well-perfused heart actually takes up lactate from the circulation and burns it to CO_2 and water. Lactate is preferred by heart muscle cells over glucose, and during endurance exercise, lactate can provide as much as 50% of your heart's energy need[28].

Liver: The liver does a whole lot of important things for the rest of the body, such as making, storing, and releasing glucose when necessary, making ketones when carbohydrate intake is restricted for more than a few days, collecting and secreting fats and lipids as lipoproteins, and making and secreting a number of important blood proteins. As a result, the liver uses a lot of energy for an organ its size, and most of the energy it uses comes from fat. The liver can get the fat it needs from circulating fatty acids released from fat cells, from remnant lipoproteins it removes from the circulation, or by making fat from carbohydrates (lipogenesis).

Brain: The brain is the spoiled child of the organ family. It can burn glucose or ketones (or a combination of the two) and it can't burn fat. This is interesting because the brain itself contains a lot of fatty acids in all its membranes and myelin (although little or none as triglycerides), and the many types of brain cells all contain mitochondria that should be capable of oxidizing fatty acids. Another surprise about the brain is how much energy it consumes each day (600 kcal) despite weighing just 3 pounds. This is more than 10-times the average energy use per pound of the rest of the body, which explains why the brain has such a large blood supply (to provide fuel and oxygen and also to keep it cool).

The other important fact about the brain's fuel supply is that it contains no reserve supply of glycogen, and because it can't burn fat, it is absolutely dependent upon a minute-by-minute blood supply containing both fuel and oxygen to meet its needs. This is why even a transient drop in blood sugar causes an intense physiological response (increased heart rate, shaking, anxiety, and intense hunger/cravings). And if blood sugar suddenly drops to less than half of the lower limit of normal, it causes coma. The shaking, anxiety, and fast heart rate that occur when blood glucose levels fall are due to a dramatic increase in adrenergic nervous system activity (release of noradrenaline from nerve endings) and adrenaline from the adrenal glands. Among other effects, this acute response to hypoglycemia stimulates two processes in liver: the breakdown of any glycogen present and formation of glucose from anything available (lactate or amino acids from protein).

Understanding this combination of facts helps explain why rapid weight loss diets, especially those emphasizing carbohydrates, can be tough to follow. If for example you decide to eat 1200 kcal per day, composed of 25% protein (75 grams), 25 % fat, and 50% carbohydrate, your daily carb intake totals just 600 kcal. That's more than enough to prevent your liver from making ketones, but it's just barely enough to feed your brain. But, you say, your liver can also make glucose from some of the protein via gluconeogenesis, which is correct, but that totals less than 50 grams (200 kcal) per day. Still, this 1200 kcal diet should support your brain's fuel needs just fine.

But what happens if you decide to go jog 5 miles in 50 minutes (which consumes 100 kcal per mile). Even at this relatively slow pace of 6 miles per hour, about half of your muscle fuel use will come from glucose or glycogen, so you burn about 250 kcal of carbohydrate fuel. In this scenario, in the 24-hours that includes this exercise, the 600 + 250 kcal of glucose use exceed the 600 + 200 kcal available supply. Typically in this setting, people start to feel lousy (see "bonking" below). Your body can make up the difference by drawing down its limited glycogen reserves or by the net breakdown of some muscle to increase liver gluconeogenesis. But if you stick to the diet and continue the daily exercise, something's got to give. And what typically happens is that your instincts (only a masochist likes to feel bad day after day) get the upper hand over your best intentions, prompting you to either eat more or exercise less.

In this situation, it would be convenient if this fuel conundrum could be solved by your liver making some ketones from body fat to help fill the gap in the brain's fuel supply. However, this appears to be a flaw in human design because liver ketone production does not kick in until daily carbohydrate intake is consistently at or under 50 grams (200 kcal) per day for a number of days. Thus there appears to be a functional gap in the body's fuel homeostasis when dietary carbohydrate intake is consistently somewhere between 600 and 200 kcal per day.

So let's consider an alternative diet, say 1200 kcal consisting of 30% protein, 15% carbs (i.e., 180 kcal or 45 grams), and 55% fat. After a week or two of getting adapted (during which you may experience some of the fuel limitation symptoms discussed above), your serum ketones rise up in the range (1-2 millimolar) where they meet at least half of the brain's fuel supply. Now if you go for that 5 mile run, almost all of your body's muscle fuel comes from fat, leaving your dietary carb intake plus gluconeogenesis from protein to meet the minor fraction of your brain's energy need not provided from ketones. And, oh yes, after your run while on the low carb diet, your ketone levels actually go up a bit (not dangerously so), further improving fuel flow to your brain.

So what does this mean for the rest of us who are not compulsive runners? Well, this illustrates that the keto-adapted state allows your body more flexibility in meeting its critical organ energy needs than a 'balanced' but energy-restricted diet. And in particular, this also means that your brain is a "carbohydrate dependent organ" (as claimed by the USDA Dietary Guidelines Advisory Committee as noted in Chapter 3) ONLY when you are eating a high carbohydrate diet. When carbohydrate is restricted as in the example above, your body's appropriate production of ketones frees the brain from this supposed state of 'carbohydrate dependency'. And because exercise stimulates ketone production, your brain's fuel supply is better supported during and after intense exercise when on a low carbo-hydrate diet than when your carbohydrate intake is high (see below).

Bonking (aka "Hitting the Wall")

Most endurance athletes know and fear a sudden loss in performance that typically occurs an hour or more into a high intensity performance. Runners call this "hitting the wall" and bicyclists call it "bonking". In either case, what the athlete describes is a common and reproducible series of events. First, no matter what else is going on around you, there is the sudden onset of food fantasies (intrusive thoughts of food). Next, within 5-10 minutes come chills and shakes (the adrenaline release). If at this point you do not immediately stop and eat, the bottom falls out of performance capacity and you feel profoundly depressed. This is why we occasionally see the highly trained runner walking the last mile of a marathon in tears. It's not just sadness from not winning – the bonked individual's brain has literally come to the bitter end of its fuel supply.

Once you know what to look for, bonking is not limited to just competition athletes. As implied above, people on energy restricted, 'balanced' (i.e., non-ketogenic) diets are quite prone to hitting the wall. And this is not limited to people doing intense exercise while on a diet. What do you think might happen to you on the above 1200 kcal 50% carb diet if you have an egg, one slice of toast (70 kcal), and unsweetened coffee for breakfast, and then a green salad and diet soda for lunch (i.e., saving 500 kcal of your allotted dietary carbohydrates for supper). At 3 in the afternoon, even if you have been sitting quietly at a desk, it is now 20 hours since your last substantial meal. What's your brain looking at for fuel? Nada.

But because this is happening when your energy expenditure is 80 kcal/hr (not 800 kcal/hr for the competing athlete), the whole process is slowed down. First the intrusive thoughts of food may last for an hour, then your anxiety and shakes come on gradually over the next half hour. In this setting, only the most stalwart person holds out against the urge to eat. If you talk to people who've been on a rigid 'balanced' diet (or perhaps remember your own experience), this is not at all an uncommon event. But if the same person restricts carbohydrate to less than 50 grams per day for a week or two, raising ketones above 1 mM, bonking disappears – whether the rapid onset version during exercise or the slow version at 3 in the afternoon.

And a final note about individual variation and bonking. Ideally everyone on a weight loss diet would not make any carbohydrate into fat (the process of lipogenesis described earlier). It stands to reason that none of the limited and precious carbohydrate intake needed to feed your brain would be "wasted" this way. However, the multiple genes that control this process have many known variants (aka polymorphisms) and thus are subject to individual variability in response to nutritional signals.

The current scientific consensus is that lipogenesis in humans is inconsequential unless they are being overfed with masses of carbohydrate. And certainly lipogenesis should be shut down during any weight loss diet when energy intake is restricted. However when we (Drs Phinney and Volek) looked for specific fatty acids produced by lipogenesis in people on low and high carb weight loss and weight maintenance diets with similar total energy contents, we saw big differences, not only between the diets, but also between individuals on the same diet[29, 30]. This implies that there is considerable inter-individual variation in the degree to which energy restriction suppresses lipogenesis. And if you are the unlucky person who still "leaks" some carbohydrate into the lipogenesis pathway during an energy-restricted 'balanced' diet, your tolerance and hence success on a "balanced" high carb weight loss diet will be impaired. This process, and the metabolic advantage associated with being keto-adapted, is further explained in Chapters 9 and 11.

For the record, the idea that lipogenesis is of any physiological importance during a weight loss diet is at best a "contrarian" position. And one might reasonably ask if any of the lipogenic enzymes have been identified as "obesity genes". But the easily identified obesity genes are those that have a strong and direct effect on food intake. However, the lipogenic pathway has a number of genes that make a number of enzymes, and a single gene effect on food intake will be subtle except under specific dietary circumstances. Thus any one of them is unlikely to stand out as an obesity gene using current methods of study, but in combination they may still have a significant effect.

Energy, Oxygen Consumption, and Respiratory Quotient (RER or RQ)

At a number of points in this text, we talk about rates of human energy use and the mix of fuels being burned. It is helpful to understand how this is measured, particularly if you want to read and be able to critique ongoing research on human energy metabolism.

The most direct method is to measure human heat production. This has been done for over a century, but even the most modern techniques are cumbersome, and they say nothing about the mix of fuels being burned (just total kcal).

The most common current method is to measure a person's oxygen consumption, and along with this, CO_2 production as well. Because carbohydrates, fats, and the carbon backbones of amino acids are all burned to CO_2 and water via the consumption of oxygen, this indirect method (called indirect calorimetry) effectively measures a person's total energy consumption.

In addition, the ratios of CO_2 produced relative to oxygen consumed are different for these three major nutrients. This ratio, the volume of CO_2 output divided by oxygen intake (VCO_2/VO_2) is 1.0 for carbohydrates, 0.70 for fat (triglyceride), and about 0.85 for protein. This ratio is called the respiratory quotient (if corrected for protein oxidation) or respiratory exchange ratio if we just use the raw number, ignoring protein metabolism. But because protein burns at 0.85, right in the middle, correcting for it tends to change the results little if at all. Thus you'll often see RQ and RER used interchangeably.

A useful rule of thumb to remember is that a liter of oxygen consumed produces about 5 kcal of metabolic energy. So a person sitting quietly reading this chapter with an energy expenditure of 1 kcal/min is consuming about 200 cc of elemental oxygen per minute (1 liter ÷ 5). If he or she had a bagel and orange juice for breakfast, most fuel being burned is glucose, so the RQ would be ~1 and CO_2 production would be about the same – 200 cc/min. However, if that person were following a very low carbohydrate ketogenic diet, O_2 consumption would be the same but CO_2 production would be a lot less, about 140 cc/min (i.e., an RQ of 0.70 is indicative of virtually pure fat oxidation).

Weight, Weight Variation, and BMI

The other set of assessment tools deserving of comment are those used to determine weight and body composition. Although modern scales are generally consistent and even pretty accurate, they suffer from not being able to differentiate water from muscle from fat. This is particularly important for the individual trying to chart her/his course on a weight loss diet because humans do not regulate their body water content precisely. So if a 70 kg adult typically contains an average of 42 liters of water, over the course of a day that person's body does not care if it contains 41 liters as opposed to 43 liters of water. Above 43 liters, the kidneys speed their function and clear the excess fluid, whereas below 41 liters, thirst prompts us to increase our water intake. The result is that most people's weight varies randomly across a range equivalent to 2 liters of water – about 4 pounds.

When humans cut back in calories, they tend to lose weight quickly at first. Some of this is water weight due to reduced glycogen reserves (the body stores 3-4 grams of water along with each gram of glycogen). But then if all subsequent weight loss comes from fat, and a 500 kcal per day deficit results in a pound per week rate of loss (assuming a pound of adipose tissue contains 3500 kcal), this weight variability within a 4 pound range can lead to a great deal of frustration and misunderstanding for the individual. This 4 pound range in weight variability could completely mask four weeks of excellent diet adherence at 1 pound per week of body fat loss. And any clinician who has worked with dieting subjects has seen individuals who are clearly sticking to much more stringent diets plateau for up to 2 weeks and then abruptly show a 5 lb weight loss. Obviously, this can be explained by the unpredictable shifts in body water content. Bottom line: the standard scale is a lousy short-term tool for monitoring your diet progress (or somebody else's diet adherence).

A relatively recent tool is the scale or device that measures weight as well as the person's electrical impedance. It is tempting to think that we can be accurately informed about total weight and total body fat content in a single measure. While these devices are useful for assessing changes in the average body composition when a large group of subjects are studied, the repetition variability for a given subject under differing conditions of temperature, hydration, and even emotional stress make it questionable for individuals as a clinical tool.

Summary

Adults can vary tremendously in body composition, ranging from 5% body fat at one extreme to 50% at the other. Lean body mass (protein containing tissue) also varies with height, gender, and physical training, but not across as wide a spectrum as body fat.

Compared to fat and protein, an adult's carbohydrate reserves are minor (ranging from a few hundred to 2000 kcal at most) and don't change that much except after extremes of exercise or food intake. When dietary carbohydrate is restricted, tissue glycogen levels decline but do not go extremely low due to compensatory shifts in whole body fuel use away from glucose towards fatty acids and ketones.

This adaptation to carbohydrate restriction is facilitated by sharply reduced insulin levels and takes a few weeks to be fully implemented. Once keto-adapted, the body can maintain its lean tissue composition on a moderate protein intake and sustain prolonged physical exertion using fat as its predominant energy supply.

Chapter 7

INSULIN RESISTANCE

Introduction

Perhaps the most important physiologic step forward in low carbohydrate diet research will come when we understand the intimate details of how insulin works in the human body and how/why normal insulin action goes awry in some individuals. Yes, that's right – we are talking about a future event here.

When Dr. Frederick Banting (a different Banting, not the undertaker who wrote the diet pamphlet) discovered insulin in 1922, for which he was awarded a Nobel Prize one year later, most people would have guessed that we'd have figured out how insulin works within a few decades. So yes, we do know that insulin binds to a receptor at the muscle cell surface, allowing glucose to be transported across the cell membrane to be used for energy or to replace depleted glycogen levels. Without the action of those glucose transporters being turned on by insulin, glucose is stuck floating around in the fluid outside of our cells. And in fat cells, stimulating the same receptor shuts off fat release and promotes fatty acid uptake, triglyceride synthesis, and fat storage.

But a big speed-bump in our understanding of how insulin works occurred in the 1930s, when scientists began observing that some people with high blood insulin levels seemed to be oblivious to its signal. Thus was born the concept of insulin resistance, broadly defined as a diminished ability of insulin to exert its normal biologic effect on a cell. And today, more than 7 decades later, we still don't fully understand the mechanism of insulin resistance – why some peoples' muscle cells just seem to thumb their noses at that big dog hormone discovered way back in 1922.

It is not that we've failed in this task for a lack of trying. As of this writing, a PubMed search on "insulin resistance" yields 57,905 citations. Hundreds of auspicious careers have been built upon the quest to understand the mechanism of insulin resistance.

So why is this important? And why waste lots of paper on a chapter whose conclusion hasn't been written yet? For one, there are several hundred million people in the world with this condition. Insulin resistance occurs on a continuum, so it's a little difficult to pin down the exact prevalence, but conservative estimates are that about 1 in 4 adults in the U.S. are insulin resistant. As with most prevalent metabolic diseases, drug companies have feverishly worked to develop pills to target the problem, but even some of the newer ones (e.g., the thiazolidine diones) as a class are running into safety problems.

The primary reason we have an entire chapter about insulin resistance is that well-formulated low carbohydrate diets consistently make it better. This benefit isn't limited to just the early phase of a low carb diet when energy intake is reduced. The improved insulin sensitivity persists for months and years into carbohydrate restriction when weight loss has ceased and most of an individual's dietary energy is coming from fat. But if you ask the average consensus expert what increasing dietary fat does to insulin sensitivity, s/he'll tell you it gets worse.

Wait a minute, you say. You tell me that low carb diets make insulin resistance get better, but then you tell me the experts say that high fat diets make it worse. How does this make sense? Are you guys prescient, or are you just one more set of charlatans selling snake oil?

Answer: we are scientists trying to figure out how the human body works. And science can't advance if we aren't ready to test out new ideas and promptly accept those that are proven to work. But part of the answer may lie in the fact that most consensus experts consider a "high fat diet" to be one with 45-60% of energy as fat, whereas we use this term for diets providing 65-85% as fat. Within our range, a well-formulated diet is almost always ketogenic, but not so in theirs. This brings us back to our analogy of that uncertain vacationer taking a flight halfway from California to Hawaii rather than committing to the whole trip. Drifting in a lifeboat halfway there is nothing like basking on the beach at Waikiki. Thus that vast body of published research using "high fat diets" in the 45-60% range for fat intake tells us nothing about what happens during nutritional ketosis. For more on this topic, see Chapter 12.

The Biology of Insulin Resistance Remains Unknown

The insulin receptor was discovered in 1969, but its 3-dimensional structure was not described until 2006. Downstream of that receptor are any number of intracellular structural pieces – like multiple rows of dominos lined up and ready to topple when insulin binds to the outside of the cell. Many of these objects (made of proteins and coded by genes) have been optimistically promoted as the cause of insulin resistance, but to no avail. None of them alone can fully explain the phenomenon of the body ignoring insulin's signal.

Part of this problem lies with how we do 'science'. The paradigm of 'modern science' is that we isolate each individual factor and study it in isolation. This is the 'reductionist' approach to discovering scientific truth. This is straight forward and relatively easy to do, so lots of scientists swear by it. But what if a clinical problem like insulin resistance is not due to a single domino, but rather a number of dysfunctional proteins or other structural materials in combination?

The answer – the reductionist approach can't deliver an answer in this situation. If multiple steps in a pathway, working in varying combinations, eventually compromise that pathway's action, the reductionist paradigm fails. But if one takes a more holistic or cosmopolitan approach to assessing the problem, the cause of the problem might be better appreciated. The rest of this chapter will offer what we think is a credible scenario that explains why and how insulin resistance gets better on a low carbohydrate diet.

Carbohydrate Increases Insulin

The primary stimulator of insulin release from the pancreas is dietary carbohydrate. In contrast, an equal amount of dietary energy as fat has virtually no effect on insulin levels. This may be obvious for educated individuals trained in nutrition and medicine, but it's worth emphasizing because it provides a theoretical construct for why a low carbohydrate diet works well in people with insulin resistance. If you consume a high carbohydrate diet, particularly one with a lot of rapidly digested sugars and refined starches, your body has an increased dependency on insulin to maintain normal metabolic homeostasis.

Specifically, the insulin released after a high carbohydrate meal is necessary to simultaneously inhibit glucose output from the liver and promote glucose uptake by skeletal muscle. Failure of insulin to perform either of these tasks, such as occurs in insulin resistance, will lead to elevated blood sugar (hyperglycemia). What this means is that when carbohydrate intake is high it puts an increased pressure on insulin to do its job effectively. If you're insulin sensitive, great - you can probably tolerate lots of carbohydrate and not run into metabolic problems. However, if insulin is struggling to perform its duties, increased consumption of carbohydrate just exacerbates an already broken system.

A low carbohydrate diet switches the body's fuel use to primarily fat. With that switch turned on, there's less need to regulate hepatic glucose output and markedly reduced surges in insulin release and glucose uptake. Thus, a low carbohydrate diet allows less dependence on insulin to maintain metabolic health. Stated another way, if we view insulin resistance as a condition of carbohydrate intolerance, dealing with dietary carbs becomes a burden, and reducing this burden allows the body to function more normally.

How is Insulin Resistance Measured?

There are a number of methods used to assess the body's response to insulin, but the definitive method is called an insulin clamp. This involves inserting multiple intravenous lines into the person, infusing insulin at a constant rate, and then measuring how much glucose has to be infused to keep the person's blood sugar constant within the normal range. The faster one needs to infuse glucose, the more sensitive that person is to the fixed dose of insulin being infused. The problem with this method is that it is complex, time-consuming, invasive, and puts the person at risk of low blood sugar (hypoglycemia) if enough sugar isn't promptly infused when needed to counteract the insulin. It is also just a measure of insulin's effects on glucose metabolism. Insulin also has an array of effects in other tissues (see Chapter 14).

A much simpler method is to simultaneously measure blood glucose and blood insulin levels and then estimate insulin sensitivity using an equation based upon insulin clamp data. For example, one of the first methods to estimate insulin resistance published in 1985 was called the homeostatic model assessment (HOMA)[31]. It is calculated as the product of fasting blood glucose x fast blood insulin divided by 22.5. Higher values indicate insulin resistance and lower values insulin sensitivity. Although these calculations of insulin sensitivity (or resistance) are just estimates, in most cases their correlation with the clamp data is reasonably good (e.g., r=0.8). While this leaves a degree of uncertainty when testing an individual, it provides a much more robust measure when assessing the response of a group of subjects to a change in diet.

Insulin Resistance is a Hallmark of Metabolic Syndrome and Type-2 Diabetes

When diabetes was first characterized as a disease a couple of centuries ago, the diagnosis was based on the appearance of sugar in the urine. This occurs only when the blood sugar level gets so high that the kidneys can't recover all of the filtered glucose, letting some of it escape into the urine.

Then doctors started measuring sugar levels in the blood, allowing earlier diagnosis. But only when the first bio-assays of insulin (followed by modern radioimmunoassay or RIA) came available could the variable response of the body to insulin be assessed.

An interesting historical note is that the publication of the first RIA of plasma insulin by Drs. Solomon Berson and Rosalyn Yalow in 1960 marked a revolution in biology and medicine eventually leading to a Nobel Prize in 1977. They distinguished two general types of diabetes: one an insulin-deficient state and the other associated with over-production of insulin.

Of the two general forms of diabetes, the clinically more dramatic form occurs when the pancreas fails to make insulin. Originally called childhood onset diabetes (because it was seen most commonly in children), this predominantly auto-immune disorder is now called type-1 diabetes. These patients need insulin injections not just to control blood glucose levels, but also to regulate the release of fats from fat cells. When fat cells release fatty acids too rapidly, ketone production becomes imbalanced and this leads to diabetic ketoacidosis. Thus ketoacidosis is characteristic of type-1 diabetes, or of late-stage type-2 diabetes that has progressed to the point that the pancreas can no longer produce the minimal amount of insulin required to limit fatty acid release from the body's fat cells.

By contrast, in most type-2 diabetics, the pancreas produces more than normal amounts of insulin because the muscle cells (which account for most of our bodies' insulin-stimulated glucose clearance) have become resistant to its signal. Typically, type-2 diabetics don't develop diabetic ketoacidosis, perhaps because their fat cells retain some of their response to insulin. This in turn helps explain why most type-2 diabetics are overweight or obese, because their fat cells are constantly maintained in storage mode by their high levels of insulin.

But insulin resistance does not develop suddenly, making yesterday's normal person into today's type-2 diabetic. It is a slow and usually silent process occurring over years or decades. As insulin resistance develops, a number of physical and biochemical changes occur. The liver turns more blood sugar into fat, so serum triglycerides go up. Fat cells spend more time in storage mode, so weight gain occurs, particularly around the center of the body, including inside the abdomen. Blood pressure also tends to rise above normal, and good (HDL) cholesterol levels go down. This combination of signs has been labeled 'metabolic syndrome', and some doctors call it pre-diabetes because a high proportion of people with 3 or more of these signs eventually develop full-blown type-2 diabetes. For more on metabolic syndrome, see Chapter 14.

Even before the signs of metabolic syndrome occur, the clever doctor/ detective can spot clues of impending diabetes. Before blood glucose and insulin start to rise; before serum triglycerides go up and HDL cholesterol goes down; before waistlines start to expand; two biomarkers of imminent trouble have been discovered. The first, a fatty acid called palmitoleic acid (POA), starts to rise in blood lipids, and it is a sign of increased conversion of carbohydrate into fat. POA is discussed in detail in Chapter 9 and also in Chapter 11. At this point, suffice it to say that an elevated level of POA in the blood is an early sign that one's body is struggling to handle whatever dose of carbohydrate is being consumed.

The second early harbinger of metabolic syndrome and type-2 diabetes is a locus of factors that we lump together under the heading 'inflammation'. Inflammation is part of what we sometimes call 'immunity' or 'host defense'. It is that complex mix of functions that our bodies use to defend against foreign substances and infections, and also how it stimulates the healing process after injury. We want inflammation levels to surge quickly when there is a threat, and retreat just as quickly when the threat is past.

About 20 years ago, it was noted that people with persistently high biomarkers of inflammation (e.g., CRP and IL-6) were at increased risk of heart attack[32, 33]. And then ten years ago this observation was extended to type-2 diabetes as well. This perspective has led us to regard inflammation as a potential underlying cause of insulin resistance and type-2 diabetes[34, 35]. Further, we now have evidence that insulin is associated with inflammation[36, 37], setting up a vicious cycle fueled by repeated ingestion of insulin-inducing carbohydrates.

Since the primary factor that drives serum insulin is dietary carbohydrate, this in turn raises the controversial possibility that dietary carbohydrate intake drives both inflammation and high blood insulin levels, both of which in turn promote insulin resistance. Does it work this way in everybody? Of course not, because we know that the other key variable is genetics. But we have just begun to scratch the surface of which genes (or gene combinations) predispose people to become 'carbohydrate intolerant'.

Dietary Carbohydrate and Its Insulin Response as Stressors of Oxidative Metabolism

This is getting pretty esoteric, so we'll keep this section short. That said, however, there are some pretty interesting dots to connect here. Inflammation causes our cells (specifically our mitochondria) to increase production of molecules called 'free radicals'. Free radicals are like mini roadside bombs that interfere with normal cellular functions. So here are the dots we think can be connected: 1) dietary carbohydrate raises serum insulin; 2) insulin promotes inflammation in susceptible people; 3) inflammation increases cellular free radical generation; 4) free radicals attack any convenient nearby target; 5) ideal targets for free radicals are membrane polyunsaturated fats; 6) membrane polyunsaturated fats are important determinants of cellular function such as insulin sensitivity.

Membrane Polyunsaturated Fatty Acids and Insulin Sensitivity

In 1993, the New England Journal of Medicine published a study demonstrating that highly unsaturated fatty acids (HUFA; e.g., arachidonate and docosahexaenoate [DHA]) in muscle membrane phospholipids are tightly correlated with insulin sensitivity[38]. Specifically, this means that the more of these HUFAs there are in the muscle membrane, the more insulin sensitive the muscle. This observation subsequently has been corroborated and extended by multiple other studies. For example the significant correlation between muscle HUFA and insulin sensitivity was shown to be specific to the phosphatidylcholine phospholipids which predominate on the outer layer of the muscle membrane[39]. This is interesting from the perspective that it implies a role for the background fatty acid composition of the membrane per se, rather than the protein components inserted into it (like insulin receptors or glucose transporters). In other words, figuratively speaking, what the 'fabric' of the wall itself is made of is very important for glucose transport – it's not just about the number of switches (i.e. receptors and transporters) inserted in the wall.

How these HUFAs get into muscle membranes is a very complex process involving both diet composition and metabolism of the various essential fats after they are eaten. This process is discussed in detail in Chapter 9. For the purposes of this chapter, both dietary intakes of either the essential fatty acid precursors or their final products are important. However, there is increasing evidence that some individuals have impaired ability to convert essential fatty acid precursors into HUFA[40].

As a rule, HUFA are a bit less prone to be burned for fuel than shorter fatty acids, so on average the body tends to hang on to them. But there is another way that they can be destroyed besides being beta-oxidized (i.e., burned for energy). As mentioned above, HUFA have lots of double bonds, and this makes them very susceptible to damage by oxygen free radicals (also called reactive oxygen species or ROS). The potential role of oxidative stress degrading membrane HUFA and thus promoting insulin resistance has yet to be fully explored, but it may be very relevant to this chapter. Here's why.

Low Carbohydrate Diets and Membrane HUFA

Twenty years ago, we published a couple of studies showing that very low calorie ketogenic diets raised the HUFA content in serum phospholipids (the building blocks for membranes)[41, 42]. The subjects for these studies started out pretty heavy and lost a lot of weight over a number of months. But after the weight loss diet was over, they went back to consuming more carbohydrate, and their HUFA levels went back down. This occurred in spite of the major weight loss, so it looked more like a diet effect than an obesity effect per se.

Recently, we have performed two more studies, one in people after 12 weeks on a low carbohydrate, high fat diet that caused a modest weight loss[29], and the second on people fed a low carbohydrate, high fat diet with sufficient calories to hold their weight stable[30]. In both cases, serum phospholipid HUFA went up when dietary carbohydrate was restricted. And also in both cases, the pattern of fatty acids in the blood did not indicate that their metabolism was making more of the HUFA – if anything, it indicated that they were making less as evidenced by consistent and marked reductions in the metabolic intermediates in their biosynthetic pathway.

In the first study, the subjects were selected because they had metabolic syndrome, so as a group, they had underling insulin resistance. After 12 weeks of the low carb diet, their insulin resistance improved by 55%, and this occurred at the same time as their blood HUFA levels were increasing. This observation does not prove that the rising HUFA levels were a direct cause of the improved insulin sensitivity, but this is certainly consistent with the observations of Borkman et al[38].

Low Carb Diets Reduce Inflammation

In the above study of people with metabolic syndrome[29], we also did a panel of tests for biomarkers of inflammation. And despite the relatively small size of the study group and the notorious variability of these biomarkers, every one of the 16 indicators of inflammation went down in the group on the low carbohydrate diet. Although some of these reductions were not statistically significant when assessed separately, the important observation is that they all went down. For that to happen purely by chance, it's like flipping a coin and getting heads 16 times in a row (which has a probability of happening once in 65,000 tries).

More importantly, that study also included a randomized comparison group given a low fat, high carbohydrate weight loss diet, and compared to their results, the low carbohydrate group had significantly greater reductions in 6 of the 16 inflammatory markers. In contrast, none of the markers were significantly lower in the low fat compared to the low carb group. In simple terms, what this means is that both energy restricted diets tended to reduce inflammation in people with metabolic syndrome, but that this effect was significantly greater with the low carbohydrate diet.

These results are consistent with other published studies comparing low carb to low fat diets. Not all low carb diet studies have shown significant reductions in biomarkers like CRP or IL-6, but many have. We suspect the variable results seen in other studies may be due to both questionable compliance with the assigned diet, plus the diets not being low enough in carbohydrate to achieve these anti-inflammatory effects.

Insulin Resistance and Diet Success

In 2007, Gardner et al published a randomized, controlled trial called the A-to-Z Study involving 4 diets lasting a year given to groups of obese women[43]. At one end of this diet spectrum was the 'Ornish diet' which is very high in complex carbs and very low in fat. At the other end was the 'Atkins diet' (i.e., low carbohydrate). After 6 months, the women on Atkins had lost significantly more weight, but after 12 months they were still lower but not significantly so. Interestingly, blood pressure and HDL cholesterol were significantly better on low carbohydrate than any of the other diets, and this beneficial effect remained significant out to 12 months.

After publishing this initial paper in JAMA, Dr. Gardner went back and examined his data based upon the subjects' insulin levels before they started dieting. When the women on each diet were divided into three subgroups (tertiles) based on baseline insulin resistance, the results were striking. In the low carbohydrate diet group, weight loss was similar in the most insulin sensitive (11.7 lbs) and insulin resistant (11.9 lbs) women. However weight loss with the high carbohydrate (Ornish) diet was much greater in the insulin sensitive (9.0 lbs) than the insulin resistant (3.3 lbs) women.

Thus the most insulin sensitive sub-groups of women experienced a similar weight loss when assigned diets either high (9.0 lbs) or low (11.7 lbs) in carbohydrate   In contrast, the sub-groups that were insulin resistant fared very poorly when assigned a diet high in carbohydrate (3.3 lbs lost) compared to a low carbohydrate diet (11.9 lbs). Specifically, those women with insulin resistance lost almost 4-times as much weight when dietary carbohydrates were restricted[44].

Simply put, insulin resistance strongly influences how we respond to different diets. This validates the concept that insulin resistance is essentially an expression of carbohydrate intolerance. Dr. Gardner's data clearly demonstrates that rather than forcing an insulin resistant body to deal with a macronutrient it can't handle well, this condition is best treated with a diet that limits carbohydrate.

Why Do Many Experts Believe that High Fat Diets Cause Insulin Resistance?

There are two general explanations for contrary data on this point. They are 1) the definition of 'high fat', and 2) the duration of the diet being tested.

The definition of a high fat diet in the scientific literature is remarkably broad. Given the current demonization of dietary fat, any diet providing more than 35% of energy as fat is typically called 'high fat'. Furthermore, most studies of humans fed 'high fat diets' go no higher than 60% of energy as fat, which means that these subjects are still getting at least 20-25% of their energy from carbohydrates. This is because the investigators either don't think the subject can tolerate a lower carbohydrate intake, or they don't think going lower on the dietary carbohydrates is safe. Of course, starting with Stefansson's Bellevue experiment, we've known for 80 years that neither of these positions is valid.

What we do know is that, pretty consistently, as dietary fat percent is increased from 30% to 60% in animals and in humans, insulin sensitivity does get worse. But once above 60% of energy as fat, which typically translates to less than 20% of energy as carbohydrates (assuming 15-20% from protein), insulin resistance turns around and starts to improve. So what's happened is that the mainstream consensus did studies of up to

60% fat, saw what looked like a straight line, and then just assumed it kept on going in a bad direction. In a word, they extrapolated themselves to a false conclusion.

But if you look at well done studies at higher fat intakes, this extrapolation doesn't stand the 'red-face test'. For example, in Dr. Guenther Boden's study of type-2 diabetics, when they cut dietary carbohydrates to 20 grams per day for just 2 weeks, there was a dramatic reduction in insulin resistance as measured by the insulin clamp technique[45]. Similarly, insulin sensitivity was dramatically improved in Dr. Forsythe's subjects with metabolic syndrome assigned to the low carb diet[29].

The other variable that can mislead us to think that high fat diets make insulin resistance worse is the duration of time on the diet. It is a common theme throughout this book that it takes humans at least 2 weeks to adapt to a low carbohydrate diet. Giving credit where credit is due, we call this the 'Schwatka imperative'. So if you read about a study where subjects were on the test diet for only a few days (or sometimes just one meal!), disregard it. Whether the parameter you are interested in is exercise performance, disposal of saturated fats, or insulin resistance, it takes at least 2 weeks of adaptation before human metabolism accurately reflects the true long-term effects of the diet.

Thus a high-fat diet is not a high-fat diet is not a high fat diet – that is to say when you read or hear someone talk about high fat diets be sure to qualify the level of carbohydrate and the period of adaptation, both of which have important effects on the outcome.

Summary

We started this chapter by telling you that the underlying cause of insulin resistance is unknown, and we finished by pointing out that low carbohydrate diets make insulin resistance better, and that insulin resistant individuals achieve more weight loss on a low carb diet compared to a very low fat diet. Clearly a great deal of science still needs to be done to explain these observations.

That said, we have also connected some very interesting dots that seem to be leading us in a consistent direction. Inflammation predicts the subsequent development of metabolic syndrome and type-2 diabetes, and inflammation is the biologic enemy of the highly unsaturated fatty acids found in cell membranes. Reduced levels of these membrane HUFAs are associated with insulin resistance, and a low carbohydrate diet simultaneously corrects the membrane HUFA deficit, improves insulin sensitivity, and reduces the body's level of inflammation.

Does this prove that insulin resistance is caused by membrane HUFA degradation as a result of inflammation and oxidative stress? Not necessarily, however it certainly makes for a strong hypothesis. But in the meantime, given the potent benefit of a well-formulated low carbohydrate diet in someone with insulin resistance, plus its very positive effects on blood lipids and fatty acids (described in the next 2 chapters), this powerful tool should not be discounted based upon ill-founded presumption, cultural bias, or extrapolated data.

Chapter 8

LIPOPROTEIN EFFECTS

Introduction

If your blood registers a high level of cholesterol, that's a surefire way to put many physicians into DEFCON mode, i.e., racing for their prescription pads. In the last decade, however, we have learned that there's much more to the heart health picture than total cholesterol. And given that this new perspective fundamentally changes our perspective on the power of dietary interventions to reduce heart disease, this chapter will attempt to explain this complex picture without the usual over-simplification.

The majority of cholesterol circulates in our bloodstream as 'low density lipoprotein cholesterol' (LDL-C), making it the prime target of drug and lifestyle strategies to prevent heart disease. While the widespread use of statins (a class of drugs used to lower cholesterol by inhibiting its production) has shown a certain degree of success in reducing cardiovascular risk, there is considerable uncertainty that cholesterol lowering per se is the primary source of this benefit. It has been argued that other mechanisms independent of reducing LDL-C (e.g., anti-inflammatory effects) may account for much of the clinical efficacy of statin drugs[46]. And yet, despite this causal uncertainty, the proposed link between blood cholesterol and heart disease has been the driving force behind dietary recommendations to restrict cholesterol and saturated fat.

But there's more to this iceberg than its obvious tip. Taken as a whole, dietary strategies to lower LDL-C have consistently failed to impact incidence of heart disease. Granted reducing cholesterol levels through diet may be an effective strategy for a subset of the population, a large number of people get no reduction in cardiovascular risk when they lower their cholesterol. If you happen to be such a person, a diet aimed at the LDL-C bull's eye not only misses the mark, it's actually aimed at the wrong target altogether.

LDL Supremacy

As the name implies, lipoproteins are spherical particles that consist of varying amounts of lipids (fat substances like cholesterol, triglycerides, phospholipids) and proteins. The lipid soluble parts are packaged in the core, whereas the water-soluble components face the periphery, thereby allowing lipoproteins to travel through the aqueous serum of the bloodstream delivering lipid cargo to and from cells. In simple terms, LDL-C (and its precursor very-low density-lipoprotein cholesterol) delivers cholesterol and other lipid substances from the liver to other organs throughout the body, whereas high-density lipoprotein (HDL-C) carries lipids in the opposite direction back to the liver for disposal. Too much cholesterol circulating as LDL-C may lead to accumulation of cholesterol in the arterial wall, plaque formation, and arterial disease.

The assumed links between high blood cholesterol and heart disease and the cholesterol-raising effects of saturated fat gained momentum between 1950 and 1970 and has been the impetus behind dietary policy for nearly four decades. However, as explained by Gary Taubes in **Good Calories, Bad Calories[13]**, rather than growing stronger as new data has accumulated over the last 40 years, the diet-heart hypothesis still stands on shaky ground. Much to the chagrin of the medical establishment and the rest of the herd defending the nutritional consensus, a growing body of literature linking low carbohydrate diets to improved lipid patterns has reached a critical mass. From a scientific perspective, the results are compelling. Nonetheless, the political situation remains that if you dare to present an alternative view opposing the tenets of the mainstream *diet-heart hypothesis,* chances are you'll be branded a heretic.

But before we get to the good stuff, we need to deal with the 800 pound gorilla in the room.

LDL Response to a Low Carbohydrate Diet

Plasma LDL-C responses to low carbohydrate diets can be variable in magnitude and direction. In well controlled experiments, the serum LDL-C level in response to a very low carbohydrate diet may increase, decrease or stay the same. In side-by-side comparison to low fat diets, LDL-C levels are usually higher in response to low carbohydrate diets[47]. This is one of the favorite talking points of low carbohydrate diet critics.

The more important question is should you be concerned if you are one of the people who show an increase in LDL-C on a low carbohydrate diet? Depending who you direct the question to, the answer may vary. Position statements and mainstream clinical guidelines recommend action steps if your serum LDL-C level is above 100 mg/dL. For most physicians, that usually means giving lip service to lifestyle changes like diet and exercise, followed promptly by a prescription for a statin drug. But let's take a minute and peel off a few more layers of the onion and consider the more balanced perspective of LDL-C offered by the research of the last decade.

First, the presumed causal link between 'total' LDL-C and heart disease is tenuous. Cholesterol reductions induced by statin drugs may be associated with reduced cardiovascular risk, but when it's a low-fat diet that lowers LDC-C, and it's compared to a higher fat diet, guess which did a better job at lowering the REAL incidence of heart disease? In 1994, the Lyon Diet Heart Study [48] was terminated prematurely at 27 months due to a dramatic decrease in mortality in the group that consumed a 40% fat Mediterranean-type diet compared to a group that was prescribed the American Heart Association's 'prudent diet'. This dramatic difference in heart disease and overall mortality occurred despite the fact that there were no differences in the two groups' LDL-C responses to the diets.

Even more convincing is the recent report from the Women's Health Initiative[49] showing that dietary fat restriction in these post-menopausal women reduced LDL-C but had **no effect** on cardiovascular disease (CVD) outcomes (heart attack, stroke, and overall mortality) after 8 years.

Second, unless your serum LDL level was determined by the more laborious direct assessment method (chances are they were not), there is potentially a high degree of error in the estimation of LDL-C (see side bar - Can You Trust Your LDL-C Numbers?).

Third, it is now well accepted that what we call LDL-C is, in fact, a complex mixture of lipoproteins consisting of particles varying across a range of sizes. Smaller LDL particles are more atherogenic (i.e., dangerous) than larger ones. And here's a key fact pertinent to this discussion: low carbohydrate diets consistently and significantly increase LDL particle size irrespective of the response in LDL-C concentration. Compelling data now indicate that having more small LDL particles is associated with increased risk for heart disease[50].

Fourth, there is a good reason serum LDL-C may transiently increase during the rapid weight loss phase of a low carbohydrate diet and it has nothing to do with the typical atherogenic theory of LDL-C (see Chapter 13).

Circling back to the question, should you be concerned if your LDL-C does not go down (or even rises slightly) on a low carbohydrate diet? In the big picture, and particularly so for people with metabolic syndrome, LDL-C is more smoke than fire. A small to moderate increase in one's total LDL-C is not worrisome if other lipid and inflammatory markers are dramatically improved in response to reducing dietary carbs. If, for example, your serum triglycerides went way down on a low carbohydrate diet (which they almost always do) then chances are you have also decreased the smaller more dangerous LDL particles even if your total LDL-C concentration increased. And as we note in the next few pages, another concurrent response to a low carbohydrate diet is increased HDL-C, which is a potent factor associated with reduced CVD risk.

Can You Trust Your LDL-C Numbers?

The most common way LDL-C is determined is to estimate its concentration using a formula derived from direct measurement of total cholesterol, HDL-C, and triglycerides. The equation was developed in 1972 by William Friedewald and colleagues[51] and continues to be routinely used in clinical assessment of cardiovascular risk and research studies, including those involving low carbohydrate diets. LDL-C is calculated as total cholesterol minus the sum of HDL-C and VLDL-C.

LDL-C = Total Cholesterol – [HDL-C + (Triglycerides/5)]

A major assumption is that the ratio of triglyceride to cholesterol is constant. VLDL is estimated as equal to triglycerides (mg/dL) divided by 5. This presumed 5:1 ratio is not constant, and the errors from this LDL-C calculation are significant[52]. In the original 1972 paper, these researchers noted that the calculation of LDL-C was inaccurate when chylomicrons were present or triglycerides were above 400 mg/dL. These essential limitations under conditions of high plasma triglycerides are widely recognized today. Less appreciated are the potential errors associated with low plasma triglycerides, a condition that is highly relevant when interpreting the LDL-C response to low carbohydrate diets since they often result in marked reductions in triglycerides.

For example, a published case report describes a man with plasma triglycerides of 55 mg/dL who had an estimated LDL-C of 172 mg/dL using the traditional Freidewald equation. But when measured by two separate direct methods, his actual LDL-C proved to be 126 mg/dL (this was also substantiated by a normal apo B level)[53]. In a formal study of 115 volunteers with plasma triglycerides less than 100 mg/dL, use of the Friedewald formula resulted in a statistically significant overestimation of LDL-C by an average of 12 mg/dL[54].

How does this play out if you are on a low carbohydrate diet? Let's assume that a low carbohydrate diet causes a reduction of triglycerides from 200 to 75 mg/dL with no change in total and HDL cholesterol. As a result, the calculated LDL-C from the Friedewald equation would necessarily increase from 100 to 125 mg/dL. How much of this 25% increase is real and how much artifact? That can only be determined by a direct assessment of LDL-C, which most physicians do not bother to do.

	TC	HDL-C	TG	LDL-C (calculated)	LDL (actual)
Before Low Carb Diet	200	60	200	100	??
After Low Carb Diet	200	60	75	125	??

LDL-C: Quality Over Quantity

Most people now have the 'LDL-C is bad and HDL-C is good' concept down pat. But there is more to the story. It is well established that not all LDL particles are created equal. Moreover, certain types of LDL have been shown to correlate with abnormal lipid profiles and promote atherosclerosis. As noted previously, the larger more buoyant LDL particles are less harmful than smaller ones. Small LDL particles reside in the circulation longer, have greater susceptibility to oxidative damage by free radicals, and more easily penetrate the arterial wall, contributing to atherosclerosis. No matter what your total LDL-C concentration, if you have relatively more small particles (referred to as Pattern B) it puts you at a several-fold higher risk for heart disease compared to people with larger LDL particles (Pattern A)[49]. And once again, this is independent of your LDL-C concentration.

How can you tell if you're pattern A or B, and how many small particles you have floating around? This is not a simple test for your doctor to do, so it's not routinely ordered by physicians, and thus it doesn't show up on standard lipid panels. The most common analytical methods use a process called gel electrophoresis, but new techniques are available based on nuclear magnetic resonance (LipoProfile Test from LipoScience) and ultracentrifugation (VAP Cholesterol Test from Atherotech).

In the mean time, the ratio of your triglyceride to HDL-C (TG/HDL-C) is an effective surrogate for LDL particle size. Values of TG/HDL-C over 3.5 indicate that you probably have pattern B with a predominance of small LDL particles, and a ratio this high indicates there's a good chance you may also have insulin resistance[55].

Statins and Low Carbohydrate Diets

Many physicians immediately turn to statins if a patient's LDL-C level is above standard guidelines, but the decision to begin lipid lowering therapy deserves serious thought. Without question statins markedly lower LDL-C but the impact on decreasing coronary events is less clear cut. For instance, the original Lipids Research Clinics (LRC) cholesterol lowering study with binding resin (cholestyramine) reduced the number of heart attacks but not overall mortality[16]. And a recent study with a statin (the JUPITER Study) indicates that much of the benefit with this class of drug is due to reduced inflammation rather than reduced LDL-C[46]. Therefore, if a diet could reduce your level of inflammation (discussed in Chapter 14), perhaps there's less need for the drug.

So in the big picture, the potential benefit of a statin drug needs to be weighed against the risk of side effects and cost of medication. The number of people who experience adverse side effects is not trivial, the most common being fatigue and muscle pain, and more recently there is concern with cognitive impairment and increased risk of diabetes. Furthermore, whether or not you make a personal or professional decision to begin statin therapy, there are still unique benefits associated with a low carbohydrate diet (see side bar – Restricting Carbohydrates has Benefits Beyond Statins).

Restricting Carbohydrates has Benefits Beyond Statins

Statin therapy effectively lowers LDL-C, but if a patient presents with other risk factors the typical course of action is to prescribe additional drugs. In the case of atherogenic dyslipidemia, combining a statin with a fibrate and/or nicotinic acid is common. While this poly-pharmacy approach can be effective in reducing lipid biomarkers, there is an increased cost and greater likelihood of side effects with multiple drug use. Importantly, in contrast to the effect of a low carbohydrate diet, none of the lipid lowering drugs are effective at reliably increasing LDL particle size. Since a low carbohydrate diet does increase LDL-C size, it represents a fully rational approach to the management of Pattern B dyslipidemia. In a research study that is currently pending publication, we examined the effect of implementing a low carbohydrate diet on LDL size and other features of metabolic syndrome in previously hyperlipidemic men and postmenopausal women who had achieved a lowered LDL-C by statin treatment. After 6 weeks the low carbohydrate diet resulted in significant improvements in a number of markers while maintaining previously reduced levels of LDL-C. LDL particle size was significantly increased as measured by two separate methods (gel electrophoresis and vertical auto profile ultracentrifugation). Additionally, there were significant improvements in plasma triglycerides (reduced by 36%), insulin sensitivity (increased by 25%), systolic (-5%) and diastolic (-6%) blood pressure, and blood flow in the forearm. In summary, atherogenic dyslipidemia and other metabolic syndrome markers are prevalent in statin users despite well-controlled LDL-C and the anti-inflammatory effects of this drug class. Thus the addition of a very low carbohydrate diet in combination with statin therapy can significantly improve insulin sensitivity, LDL quality, and other features of metabolic syndrome.

In summary, if LDL-C is your sole intended target, a low fat diet and/or cholesterol-lowering drugs appear to make sense. But there is enough doubt to question whether LDL-C is the best target for everyone. If your target encompasses a broader range of potent biomarkers like triglycerides, HDL-C, LDL particle size, insulin resistance, or inflammatory markers, then using a low fat/high-carbohydrate diet is equivalent to dancing on the edge of a mine field, whereas a low carbohydrate diet improves all these blood borne risk markers[56].

Triglyceride as a Target

The reductionist focus on total LDL-C as the only valid therapeutic target has distracted us from the mounting evidence that other biomarkers may be better predictors of risk, especially if you (or your patient) have insulin resistance. If LDL-C is not the most relevant target for many people, what is? Many studies have reported that an elevated fasting plasma triglyceride level is an independent risk factor for heart disease. If you have high triglycerides after an overnight fast, there is a good chance you also have elevated postprandial lipemia (an exaggerated and prolonged increase in plasma triglycerides after a meal).

Abnormal postprandial lipemia is the driving force behind the dyslipidemia of the atherogenic lipoprotein phenotype (ALP). ALP is a term frequently used to describe a clustering of pro-atherogenic lipoprotein abnormalities including moderately increased fasting triglycerides (150 to 500 mg/dL), exaggerated postprandial lipemia, decreased HDL-C (<40 mg/dL), and a predominance of atherogenic small dense LDL particles (pattern B).

These lipid disorders have also been referred to as the 'lipid triad' or 'atherogenic dyslipidemia'. The prevalence of ALP varies depending on the criteria used (i.e., triglyceride, HDL level, or LDL size). When defined as peak LDL particle diameter <25.5 nm, ALP has been estimated at a prevalence of 30-35% in middle-aged men in the United States. So what makes having high post-prandial triglycerides harmful? Increased hepatic triglyceride production precipitates formation of highly atherogenic small LDL particles and a reduction in HDL cholesterol, all of which indicate a causal role for elevated triglycerides in the pathogenesis and progression of heart disease.

Carbohydrate is the Major Driver of Plasma Triglycerides

An increase in fasting triglyceride levels is an early signal that your body is struggling to metabolize carbohydrate. Therefore the weapon of choice for managing elevated triglyceride levels is carbohydrate restriction. Why restrict carbs and not fat? Most people have a total of about 20 grams (a little more than 1 tablespoon) of extra-cellular glucose – 10 grams circulating in their blood and another 10 grams diffused into extra-cellular fluid. A single meal from a 'balanced diet' can easily contain well over 100 grams carbohydrate, necessitating a mechanism to rapidly dispose of the incoming carbohydrate in order to maintain normal blood glucose. In the resting state much of this glucose should be converted to glycogen in skeletal muscle and liver. However, these organs have a maximum storage capacity of about 400 and 100 grams, respectively.

In addition to this limited capacity to store carbohydrate in the body, the metabolic conversion of glucose to glycogen (glycogen synthesis) is relatively slow, and in particular it is markedly impaired in individuals with insulin resistance. How then does a person with insulin resistance deal with a high carbohydrate meal? Whereas the conversion of glucose to glycogen is self-limiting, there is an almost infinite capacity to convert carbohydrate to fat (aka, de novo lipogenesis). The fatty acids derived from carbohydrate-induced hepatic de novo lipogenesis are made into triglycerides, packaged into large VLDL particles, which are then released into the circulation, contributing to elevated plasma triglycerides. Alternatively, if they are not released from the liver, these triglycerides can build up to cause fatty liver (hepatic steatosis).

Carbohydrate is the Major Driver of LDL Particle Size

The formation of LDL particles of varying sizes is intimately linked with triglyceride metabolism in the liver. When viewed through metabolic binoculars, it comes as no surprise that dietary carbohydrate has a predictable effect on LDL size. Dietary carbohydrate restriction increases the prevalence of larger LDL particles, whereas low fat/high carbohydrate diets have the opposite (and overtly harmful) effect. This inverse relationship between dietary carbohydrate content and LDL size is evident over a wide range of carbohydrate intakes[57], and it can have quite dramatic (i.e., positive) effects at very low carbohydrate intakes[56]. As people move down the carbohydrate ladder, more and more of them convert their serum lipids from pattern B to Pattern A and thus decrease their cardiovascular risk. And moving up the carbohydrate continuum has the opposite effect. In carefully controlled feeding studies, low fat/high-carbohydrate diets decrease LDL particle size, causing some individuals to shift from pattern A to pattern B[58, 59].

The Triglyceride Saturated Fat Connection

An additional highly relevant aspect of plasma triglyceride is its fatty acid composition. Blood triglycerides containing saturated fatty acids are more highly correlated with insulin resistance than ones containing essential fatty acids[60]. In addition, a number of prospective and case-controlled studies associate higher proportions of saturated fats in blood lipids with increased coronary disease risk[61-63]. How does one come to have more saturated fat in their blood lipids? If you subscribe to the simplistic concept that you are what you eat, then you might believe that dietary saturated fats are to blame for insulin resistance and coronary disease.

However association does not prove causality. The alternative explanation is that an insulin resistant liver readily converts carbohydrate to fat (de novo lipogenesis), and the main product of this pathway is the saturated fat palmitic acid (16:0). When stressed by excess dietary carbohydrate, the liver secretes highly saturated triglyceride-rich VLDL particles. Once in the circulation, these large VLDL are readily converted to small atherogenic LDL particles. Having a lot of saturated fat in your triglycerides, therefore has little to do with your dietary saturated fat intake, but rather how much carbohydrate you eat and how effectively (or ineffectively) your body processes it (see side bar and also Chapter 9).

Dietary Carbohydrate: Saturated Fat's Evil Twin

Saturated fat in the diet gets blamed for a lot of bad things. It turns out most of the harmful effects attributed to dietary saturated fat (e.g., increased heart disease, insulin resistance, vascular dysfunction, etc.) are unsubstantiated. The truth is that saturated fats only become problematic when they accumulate. And the guilty party for saturated fat accumulation, in most cases, is dietary carbohydrate.

Yes; dietary intake of carbohydrate - not saturated fat - is the major driver of plasma levels of saturated fat. Counter-intuitively, prior studies have reported lower plasma levels of saturated fat in response to diets that contained 2-3 fold greater intake of saturated fat but were lower in carbohydrate[29, 64, 65]. Even in controlled feeding studies in weight stable individuals (which necessitates a high intake of dietary fat), low carbohydrate diets decrease plasma saturated fat levels[30].

A cautious reader might suggest that the saturated fats are not show- ing up in our tests because they are leaving the blood and accumu- lating in tissue triglycerides. But we have done this experiment in mice adapted to a low carbohydrate diet, and despite eating almost 3-times as much saturated fat as the control mice for 8 weeks, tis- sue levels of saturates are the same or lower in the low carb mice. How can this be? Clearly, humans and mice adapted to a low car- bohydrate diet by becoming very adept at using saturated fats as the preferred fuel in muscles and liver. Thus, from the body's perspective, a low carbohydrate diet reduces both blood and tissue saturated fat levels irrespective of dietary saturated fat intake.

Importance of Raising HDL-C

HDL-C is one of the best biomarkers of long term cardiovascular health. Unfortunately for drug companies, however, it is a therapeutic target for which existing drugs have little efficacy. Low levels indicate significant cardiovascular risk independent of LDL-C. The importance of HDL-C derives from its well established role as a scavenger of excess unesterified cholesterol from lipoproteins and tissues requiring transport back to the liver (i.e., reverse cholesterol transport).

HDL-C also increases bioavailability of nitric oxide (important to the regulation of vascular function and blood pressure) and has antioxidant, anti-inflammatory, anti-thrombotic, and anti-apoptotic effects, all of which contribute to its antiatherogenic properties. Almost as consistent as their triglyceride-lowering effects, low carbohydrate diets increase HDL-C[47]. The increase in HDL-C may not occur as quickly as the decrease in triglyceride, but based on empirical evidence and the results of a recent 2 year diet study[66], this slowly developing HDL-C boost appears to be very resilient. A notable feature of this study was the gradual increase in carbohydrates over the 2 year intervention which in this case resulted in a concomitant loss of the triglyceride-lowering benefit but a persistent benefit in HDL-C.

	Diet	Diet Intervention			
		3 mo	6 mo	12 mo	24 mo
Change Triglyceride	Low Carb	-35%	-35%	-28%	-11%
	Low Fat	-15%	-20%	-14%	-12%
Change HDL-C	Low Carb	5%	13%	17%	17%
	Low Fat	-1%	2%	9%	10%

Summary of lipid responses (percent change from baseline [66]).

The Triglyceride/HDL Ratio as a Correlate to Insulin Resistance

In the search for lipoprotein markers that correlate with insulin resistance and predisposition to CVD, recent research has focused on the ratio of triglyceride/HDL-C. Studies indicate the triglyceride/HDL-C ratio is highly associated with insulin resistance[55]. Simply put, the higher your triglycerides and/or the lower your HDL-C, the greater your degree of insulin resistance. This association was stronger than any other lipid parameter and was equal to that of the more conventional methods using fasting glucose and insulin such as the Homeostasis Model Assessment of Insulin Resistance (HOMA-IR) and Quantitative Insulin Sensitivity Check Index (QUICKI). The ratio is comparable to the ATP III criteria for metabolic syndrome in predicting insulin resistance and even better in prediction of the LDL Pattern B phenotype in two separate populations who were on different diets. A TG/HDL ratio ^{3}3.5 has been suggested as a cutoff for identifying the insulin-resistant patient most at risk for cardio-vascular disease[55].

Summary

The syllogistic logic that reducing dietary saturated fat intake decreases LDL-C concentration, which in turn decreases heart disease, has come under severe scrutiny. There is a growing recognition that replacing fat with carbohydrate has untoward negative effects on non-LDL lipid parameters, such as serum TG and HDL-C. We have examined the strengths and limitations of LDL-C with its Pattern A and B variants, HDL-C, and triglycerides as biomarkers of risk, and pointed out the differing effects of low fat and low carbohydrate diets on each. The triglyceride /HDL ratio provides a broader assessment of risk, and its relationship with insulin resistance makes it far superior to LDL-C.

And how best to improve your triglyceride/HDL ratio? The striking reductions in plasma triglycerides and consistent increases in HDL-C in response to low carbohydrate diets are unparalleled by any other lifestyle intervention, or even drug treatment, and therefore represents the most powerful method to improve this ratio. These lipid parameters may be more important targets as they reflect how efficiently the body is processing dietary carbohydrate and the level of insulin resistance. This is described in greater depth in Chapter 14.

Post-Script: Triglyceride Metabolism Primer

Chemically, a triglyceride is composed of 3 molecules of fatty acids bound to a glycerol backbone. Triglyceride is the major type of fat ingested and stored in the body. Food containing triglycerides are digested primarily in the small intestine and then re-esterified back to triglycerides and packaged into chylomicrons within intestinal cells. Chylomicrons enter the circulation via the lymphatic system. Triglycerides are also made in the liver and packaged into lipoproteins called very low density lipoproteins (VLDL) that are released into the plasma. Chylomicrons and VLDL therefore constitute the triglyceride-rich lipoproteins. The liver synthesizes apo-B-100 which associates with VLDL, whereas the intestine synthesizes an abbreviated version apo-B-48 that associates with chylomicrons. The triglycerides in chylomicrons and VLDL are hydrolyzed by lipoprotein lipase (LPL) located in the capillary walls of various tissues, primarily skeletal muscle and adipose tissue. The primary functions of LPL are to clear triglycerides from the circulation and augment the supply of free fatty acids to various tissues such as skeletal muscle, adipose tissues, and heart for either storage or oxidation. Both chylomicrons and VLDL contain apo-C-II, which is required as a cofactor for LPL activity. After nearly complete hydrolysis of the triglycerides, the remaining portion is referred to as a chylomicron or VLDL remnant. These remnant lipoproteins are relatively rich in cholesterol and cholesteryl esters and retain their apo-E and apo-B proteins, however apo-C is transferred to nascent (newly formed) HDL-C. Uptake of chylomicron and VLDL remnant lipoproteins occurs via specific receptors on the liver which recognize apo-E and apo-B-100 proteins, respectively. Chylomicron remnants are taken up directly by the apo-E receptor, whereas VLDL remnants are first converted into an intermediate density lipoprotein (IDL), which in turn may be either converted into LDL or be taken up by the liver via the apo-B-100/E receptor.

Chapter 9

EFFECTS OF CARBOHYDRATE RESTRICTION ON FATTY ACID METABOLISM

Introduction

Part of the human body's adaptation to carbohydrate restriction involves fundamental changes in how it metabolizes fatty acids. Of course it makes sense that stopping most of your dietary carbohydrate intake will force the body to speed up its rate of total fat oxidation. But there's much more to this story than that.

Not only does total fat oxidation increase, but the body's rate of saturated fat oxidation accelerates more than other types of fatty acids, driving down levels of saturated fat in the blood. Also, the body literally stops making fat out of carbohydrate (i.e., de novo lipogenesis), much of which ends up as saturated fats in the blood. Understanding that this happens and why opens an important door to our understanding of how a high fat diet, even one containing a lot of saturated fat, can still be healthy.

But perhaps equally (if not more) important is the dramatic change in how our bodies handle polyunsaturated fats when we cut back on carbohydrate intake. Polyunsaturates are obligate components of phospholipids, which in turn are needed to construct the membranes that enclose our cells and regulate cellular functions. Getting the right amount of polyunsaturated fats into membranes is critical for life-defining processes such as glucose transport (i.e., insulin sensitivity), controlling inflammation, salt excretion, blood pressure control, egg release from ovarian follicles, and sperm motility.

Disposing of a Myth

We've all heard the saying "you are what you eat". Mothers and spouses love to tell us this when we are eating something 'bad'. Unfortunately, within the realms of dietetics and medicine, this oft-repeated aphorism has become synonymous with the truth. Why is this unfortunate? Because it's not true.

A typical lean, healthy human eats ten times as many calories per year as s/he has in body energy stores. So over a decade, that translates to about 99% of what we eat getting burned. And at many levels in the processes of digestion, absorption, transport, storage, and oxidation, the body has a choice of what it saves and what it burns.

So the true aphorism is "you are only that very small fraction that your body chooses to save from what you eat".

Which means you can eat Twinkies without becoming one, or eat beef without growing horns.

Getting back to the topic of fat metabolism, this means that your body has a remarkable ability to select what it wants to keep while burning off the rest. It also means that you can selectively store specific fatty acids in specific places. Thus the mix of fats found in membrane phospholipids is dramatically different from that found in the triglycerides stored in adipose tissue. And even the mix of fatty acids in our adipose tissue triglycerides varies from site to site. For example, the fat composition in your legs is different from the mix found around your abdomen[67]. So the next time you hear someone argue a point by stating "you are what you eat", be sure to treat that person's opinion with a healthy dose of skepticism.

Disposing of Saturated Fats

There are three things we can do with saturated fats obtained from, or produced as a result of, our diet: burn them, store them, or make them into something else (e.g., a mono-unsaturate). Insulin, which goes up in the blood when we eat carbohydrates, turns off fat oxidation and stimulates fat storage. And when we stop eating lots of carbs and our insulin levels fall, the opposite happens; fats come out of storage and become the body's primary fuel.

But what happens if you eat more total grams of saturated fat when you stop eating all those carbohydrate calories? This comes down to an issue of balance. Which side wins - the increased intake of saturated fats or their increased oxidation in the keto-adapted individual? The answer is not obvious because we now know that our metabolism has the capability to differentiate between types of fat based on chain length and number of double bonds.

To answer this question, we took blood samples from twenty people after 12 weeks on a low carbohydrate diet and another twenty who had been following a low fat, high carb weight loss diet[29]. In the serum from both groups, we measured both total triglyceride and its specific fatty acid composition. But before we tell you what we found, we also need to tell you that the saturated fat intake of the low fat diet group was 12 grams per day, while the low carbohydrate group was eating 36 grams per day – three times as much.

In the serum samples done at baseline and again after 12 weeks, serum triglycerides in the low fat group went from 187 to 151 mg per 100 ml, a tidy 19% reduction. But in the low carb group, the before and after values were 211 and 104, a whopping 51% fall. Both visually (just looking at the numbers) and statistically, the low carbohydrate group had a much greater (better) reduction in serum triglycerides.

But what about the fatty acids contained in this serum fraction? As a proportion of the total, the low carb group had 33% saturates at baseline and 29% after 12 weeks, whereas the low fat group started at 30 and ended at 29%. So after 12 weeks of dieting, the proportion of saturated fats in the blood triglycerides was the same for both groups despite the fact that the low carb group was eating three times as many grams per day of saturated fat in their diet.

But there's more. Because the low carb group ended up with blood triglycerides of 104 mg per 100 ml compared to the low fat group's 151, they actually had about 30% less total triglycerides circulating in their serum. So although the two groups had similar relative proportions of saturates, this means that the absolute serum content of saturates in the low carb group was 30% lower than the low fat diet group. So what we found, in a nutshell, is that despite a higher intake of saturated fat, the proportionate blood level of saturated fats did not increase, and their absolute levels fell dramatically with the low carbohydrate diet.

Now, it's fair to ask, what about other parts of the body like the liver, muscles, and fat cells. Maybe all that saturated fat from the diet is just getting tucked away and doing bad things somewhere other than in the blood. Well, that isn't likely given the low insulin levels associated with a low carbohydrate intake. But to check this issue in a group of subjects that were willing to let us take pieces of their muscle, liver, and fat to examine, we put some mice on these two diets.

After 8 weeks, during which the low carb mice ate two and a half times as much saturated fat, in 4 tissues examined, the triglyceride content of saturated fats was either the same (soleus muscle and liver) or significantly reduced (gastrocnemius muscle and adipose tissue [aka fat cells]) in the low carb group compared to the low fat group.

The bottom line on this point is that when our metabolism adapts to a low carbohydrate diet, saturated fats become a preferred fuel for the body, and their levels in blood and tissue triglyceride pools actually drop. There are currently valid questions being raised about whether dietary saturated fat intake represents any health risk at all, even in people who eat modetare amounts of dietary carbohydrate. But clearly, in the context of a keto-adapted individual following a low carbohydrate diet, where saturated fat disposal is accelerated causing blood levels to drop, there is no basis to be concerned about their inclusion in the foods we choose to eat.

Making Fat from Carbohydrate – The POA Story

We humans have all of the cellular machinery needed to make carbohydrates into fat, concentrated mostly in liver and fat cells. But for the past 2 decades, the consensus experts have dictated that this becomes important in humans only when one's intake of carbohydrate calories exceeds the body's total rate of energy use. This position is supported by a great deal of scientific data, but it stands up only if one makes a lot of assumptions. One of those assumptions is that most of the fat made by our cells remains as the saturated fat palmitate (16 carbons with no double bonds). But we believe that assumption is not correct, and here's why.

Fifteen years ago, we did a study at UC Davis where we fed a group of women all their food for 4 months. For that whole time, each person was fed just enough total calories to keep her weight stable. But what changed over those 4 months was that we progressively reduced their fat intake from 31% to 25%, and then to 15%. At each step, when we took away fat calories, we added an equal amount of carbohydrate while holding protein intake constant.

And to keep the diet as healthy as possible, the added carbohydrates were in the form of complex starches and grains, keeping total sugar intake as low as possible. In spite of this, serum triglycerides rose progressively as the fat was removed from the diet[68]. And when we looked at the blood fatty acids, the proportion of palmitate and total saturates were significantly increased. But the biggest proportionate change in any of the serum fatty acids was a mono-unsaturated 16-carbon fatty acid called palmitoleic acid (POA, technical abbreviation 16:1w7[see Figure 2 Page 117]). Among fatty acids attached to cholesterol in the serum (called cholesteryl esters, or CE), POA almost doubled as dietary fat was reduced from 31% to 15%.

POA is what the body makes from palmitate using the enzyme SCD1 (explained in post-script at end of chapter), and POA was clearly identified as a major product of human lipogenesis in 1998[69]. In that study, the subjects were fed massive doses of carbohydrates. But in our study at UC Davis, the subjects weren't being overfed, so based on prevailing assumptions about lipogenesis, they weren't "supposed" to be making much of their dietary carbohydrate into fat. But our test subjects, at a stable weight, did have progressively increased serum POA as dietary fat was replaced by carbohydrate. And to be sure this wasn't just happening in the blood; we also took small bits of body fat using a needle, and we found POA accumulating in their adipose tissue triglycerides as well.

But what was most interesting about POA in these subjects was how much they differed one from another. After a month on the 31% fat diet when everyone had been eating exactly the same food, the serum CE POA ranged from 2% to 6%. Three months later, after 6 weeks eating 15% fat, serum POA now ranged from 3% to 10%. Of the 28 subjects in the study, two had no change in their CE POA as they ate more and more carbohydrate in place of fat, but among the other 26, all of their POA values went up. And they seemed to do it in parallel – those who started low went up modestly, whereas those who started high went up more rapidly. This implies that there is a lot of diversity among healthy humans in how much POA they make (and perhaps total conversion of dietary carbs to fat) under standardized dietary conditions. And it also indicates that we can use POA as a biomarker for lipogenesis.

This concept of POA as a biomarker of carb conversion to fat was further reinforced when we looked at POA in the subjects from our recent study of people put on a low carb diet for 12 weeks[29]. In addition to the saturated fat data noted earlier in this chapter, we also looked at POA levels in their serum CE fraction. In this case, our baseline data was obtained when they were eating 36% of their energy as fat, and the second sample came after eating 59% from fat. These samples, plus the high carb feeding study mentioned above, are presented together in Figure 1. This shows again that there was more diversity in POA between subjects at 36% than at 59% dietary fat, and that the group as a whole came down dramatically at the higher fat intake.

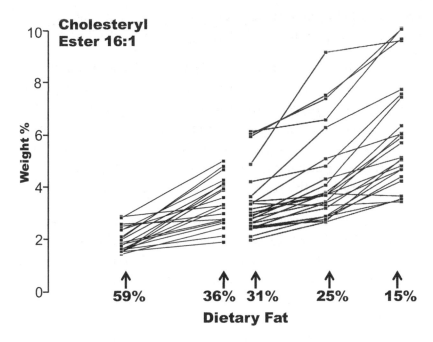

Figure 1. Cholesteryl ester palmitoleic acid (aka CE POA).
Proportion expressed as wt% versus % dietary fat from two study cohorts.

So what do we know about POA, and is it really important enough to jus-tify struggling through all this detail? Well, it has been observed that se-rum POA predicts the subsequent development of type-2 diabetes. In two published studies, people without any increase in blood sugar levels but increased POA are at high risk of becoming diabetic later on[70, 71]. The consensus experts don't seem to know why this happens, but from our research perspective, it looks like increased POA levels are a sign that the body is having difficulty getting glucose into muscle cells to be burned. As an alternative, glucose is diverted to fat production in the liver just to get rid of it, and this starts happening long before blood sugar levels rise.

But stepping back just a bit, POA functions a bit like Galileo's telescope. As he watched the moons of Jupiter go around that big planet, Galileo realized that the Earth and its moon were similarly revolving around the sun. So what's the 'eureka moment' that comes from looking at POA levels? If some apparently healthy people eating more than 20% of their energy from carbs make a lot of POA, and this increases as the carbohydrate dose increases, then who's the 'perp' in this crime? Hello? It's all about the carbs!

As we noted above, POA predicts insulin resistance and type 2 diabetes. Reducing carbohydrate reduces serum POA levels. People with type 2 diabetes who restrict carbs get better or even go into complete remission. But two individuals at the same level of carb intake can differ greatly in how much POA they make, so it stands to reason that diets need to be adjusted to the tolerances of each individual. Forget about the idea that "one diet is perfect for everyone". This issue is discussed in greater detail in Chapter 11.

Bottom line: POA is a sensitive (and powerful) biomarker of carbohydrate intolerance. Long before classic signs of diabetes (high blood sugar, elevated hemoglobin A1c) develop, POA goes up. This is a tool that could tell the clinician who is at risk well before other indicators. And once these people are identified, POA might be used to guide each individual to the right level of carbohydrate restriction to keep this problem in remission. Unfortunately POA is still a research test that is not standardized and available to clinical practitioners, but we hope this test will be made available in the near future.

The Polyunsaturated Fatty Acid Response to Carbohydrate Restriction

Most serious scientists avoid the topic of polyunsaturated fatty acid (PUFA) metabolism like a plague. Why? Because it's a tangle of obscure names and symbols, parallel metabolic pathways, and positional isomers with conflicting functions. And besides, there are so many of them! In a single serum fraction, we typically identify about 20 different fatty acids with two or more double bonds (the definition of a polyunsaturate) belonging to 3 different metabolically distinct families (for details, see post-script below).

So again, it is fair to ask, what's the upside of opening this metabolic can of worms? The answer, simply, is that the dramatic changes in PUFA associated with adapting to a low carbohydrate diet can help explain the underlying physiology of its benefits.

First, we'll offer you an overview of why that might be. Then we'll tell you how we stumbled into this understanding over the last 20 years.

Point 1. Low carbohydrate diets cause the physiologically important end-products of essential fatty acid (EFA) metabolism in membranes to go up sharply[29, 41, 42]. EFA end-products in muscle membranes are positively correlated with insulin sensitivity[38]. Thus these membrane composition changes can explain the improved insulin sensitivity that occurs when an insulin resistant individual adopts a low carbohydrate diet.

Point 2. Increased EFA end-products in liver membranes shut down expression of the enzymes that drive lipogenesis[72]. The consensus experts assume that human lipogenesis is inconsequential, however, they see no reason to explain how it stops when dietary carbs are reduced. But from the perspective offered by POA, something clearly puts the brakes on lipogenesis when a person transitions to a low carbohydrate diet, and our observation of increased EFA end-products offers an elegant mechanism. In addition, this helps explain the dramatic reduction in serum triglycerides that we see in individuals with metabolic syndrome who go on a low carbohydrate diet.

Point 3. A simple explanation for increased EFA end-products might be that the body makes more of them on a low carb diet. But unfortunately it isn't that simple. All of the data (levels of metabolic intermediates and enzyme activities) point in the opposite direction – that production of EFA end-products goes down! So if they go up without more being made, this indicates that the body must be destroying them more slowly. And since the arch-enemy of PUFA is a group of molecules we call free-radicals (or more precisely, reactive oxygen species – ROS), perhaps the rate of ROS generation is reduced when dietary carbohydrates are restricted. The mainstream consensus still regards this as an 'outside the box' (or should we say "radical") fantasy, but it is also consistent with our multiple observations that a host of biomarkers of inflammation (known inducers of ROS generation) go down when a low carb diet is adopted[29].

So there you have it. It's really kind of elegant. Inflammation driven by the forced metabolism of carbohydrate drives up the production of ROS in mitochondria. ROS damage membrane EFA end-products, which at some point can't be replaced fast enough. The resultant reduction in membrane EFA end-products unleashes the genes (e.g. fatty acid synthase) that control liver lipogenesis, and at the same time the loss of membrane HUFA causes increased insulin resistance in muscles. Insulin resistant muscles take up less glucose, resulting in more of it being diverted to the liver for lipogenesis. Take away the high levels of ROS and membranes suffer less damage, their content of EFA end-products rises, and both dyslipidemia and insulin resistance improve. The trigger for this set of metabolic dominos – the switch that controls this process – is dietary carbohydrate.

Summary

Clearly there is much more to dietary fats and health than is contained in simplistic edicts like "saturated fats are bad for you". We have shown you that our bodies respond to saturated fats very differently when we are keto-adapted, such that they are rapidly burned for fuel rather than being stored. By contrast, people eating higher levels of dietary carbohydrates, even when they are not over-eating total calories, have higher blood levels of saturated fats. As illustrated by the elevated levels of POA associated with higher proportions of dietary carbohydrate, some individuals are particularly prone to dispose of dietary carbohydrates via lipogenesis, which creates a lot of saturated fatty acids as well as POA.

The other new and important insight into the fatty acid response to carbohydrate restriction comes from examining the changes in EFA end-products in phospholipids. Keto-adaptation results in marked changes in how our bodies are able to construct and maintain optimum membrane composition, and this appears to be due to less production of ROS and inflammatory mediators. There is much more for us to learn about this process, but at the very least, this observation helps explain the improvement in insulin sensitivity that occurs when you become keto-adapted.

Post-script: Details of Fatty Acid Nomenclature and Metabolic Pathways

This section is included here for the reader who wants more detail about the names and metabolic relationships among the various types (classes) of fatty acids. If you haven't taken chemistry or biochemistry in the past (or if you didn't enjoy it), you might decide to skip this section and move on to the next chapter. But for many readers, working through this section will facilitate your understanding of a number of points we make about fats and fatty acid metabolism elsewhere in this book.

Fatty acids are generally classed by the length of the carbon chain – 'short' (2, 3, or 4), 'medium' (6 to 12) and 'long' (14 or more) – and by the number of double bonds within that chain. Saturated fats have no double bonds, mono-unsaturates have one double bond in the carbon chain, and polyunsaturates have two or more double bonds.

Short-chain fatty acids are commonly consumed in the diet, such as acetic acid (2-carbons) in vinegar and lactic acid (3 carbons) in yogurt, buttermilk, natural cheese and some fermented vegetable products like saukraut and kimchi. In addition, the 'ketones' made in our liver – beta-hydroxybutyrate and acetoacetate – are 4 carbon fatty acids which, like lactate, have an extra oxygen attached to the carbon chain. All of these, whether consumed in the diet or produced metabolically, are rapidly oxidized as fuel by a variety of tissues as described in Chapter 6.

Medium-chain fatty acids are found in dairy fats (milk, butter and cream) and in some 'tropical oils' like palm oil. These fatty acids, with the slight exception of 12-carbon laurate, are not incorporated into triglycerides and stored in the body. Once eaten, they must be promptly oxidized for fuel by mitochondria. Unlike long-chain fatty acids that require assistance from mitochondrial membrane proteins to get into the mitochondrial matrix, medium-chain fatty acids bypass this regulatory step. If we consume more medium-chain fats than can be burned in a short period of time, our liver converts the excess into ketones, which in turn can be burned by a wider range of organs (e.g., the brain).

Long-chain fatty acids consumed in the diet can be either oxidized (burned for energy) or stored as triglycerides. As a general rule, the longer the carbon chain, the more likely a fatty acid is to be stored. But this is not uniformly true, because an unsaturated fatty acid with a double bond close to the 'omega-end' (the opposite end of the chain from the terminal 'COOH' carboxylic acid moiety) is more likely to be oxidized than a chain of equal length with any double bonds farther away from the omega-end[73]. Thus omega-3 fatty acids, which are so named because they have a double bond that is just 3 carbons from the omega-end, are more readily oxidized for fuel than analogous omega-6 or omega-9 fatty acids. These differing metabolic preferences for oxidation over storage help explain why the composition of our body fat stores differs from the composition of the fats in our diet (i.e., why we aren't what we eat).

Among the polyunsaturated fatty acids, there are two sub-groups that are essential for human well-being and function. These consist of two separate families each ranging in chain length from 18 to 22 carbons. The omega-6 family, all having a double bond 6-carbons in from the omega-end, starts with its 18-carbon precursor linoleate (18:2ω6) and can be elongated and desaturated to a series of products which all retain the original omega-6 double bond. For the most part in human metabolism, this process stops with arachidonate (20:4ω6). This series of steps is depicted vertically on the left side of the Figure 2. Note also that this numerical short-hand consists of the number of carbons (e.g., for arachidonate 20), following the colon is the number of double bonds (4), and the ω6 indicates the distance from the first double bond to the omega-end. All additional double bonds occur at 3-carbon intervals.

These same enzymes that process omega-6 fatty acids also elongate and desaturate the omega-3 precursor alpha-linolenate (18:3ω3 – not to be confused with linoleate – which is why the numerical 'omega' shorthand is better). However rather than stopping with the omega-3 product EPA (20:5ω3) which is analogous to arachidonate, most of the omega-3 product found in human tissues is docosahexaenoate (22:6ω3, or DHA for short). Even people who eat a lot of fish or fish oil supplements, which contain lots of EPA, still have more DHA than EPA in their cell membranes. Thus this pathway with its various FADS and elongase enzymes actively processes what we eat to try and maintain the optimum collection of 'essential fatty acid end products' like arachidonate and DHA in our cell membranes.

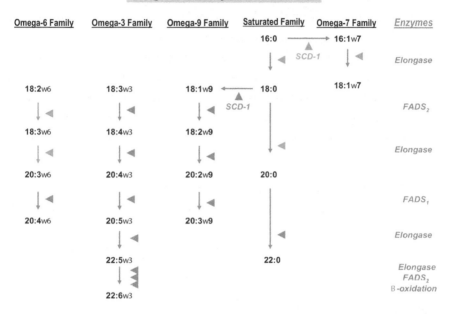

Long-chain Fatty Acid Anabolism

Figure 2. Enzymatic metabolism of essential (omega-6 and omega-3) and non-essential fatty acid families. SCD-1, steroyl-CoA-desaturase, adds a double bond 9-carbons in from the acid end of the carbon chain. FADS$_2$, fatty acid desaturase-2, adds a double bond 6-carbons in from the acid end. FADS$_1$ adds a double bond 5-carbons in from the acid end. Elongase adds two carbons to the chain at the acid end. Because all of these enzymes work at the acid end, an omega-3 or omega-6 double bond does not change in relation to the omega-end when these additions are made at the other end of the chain. Thus an omega-3 fatty acid remains an omega-3 fat until it gets burned for fuel, and the same goes for the omega-6 family. Metabolically, they cannot be inter-converted (which is why there are no horizontal arrows on the left side of this figure. SCD-1, on the other hand, can add a double bond to a saturated fat, making either an omega-9 mono-unsaturate (oleate, 18:1ω9) if starting with 18:0, or palmitoleate (POA, 16:1ω7) when starting from 16:0.

An important point that we touch on a number of times in this book is that when a person switches from a high carb diet to one low enough in carbohydrate that the body starts making ketones (usually at or under 50 grams per day of total carbs), the body's economy of essential fatty acids changes dramatically. This is seen as a rise in both arachidonate and DHA in serum phospholipids, while at the same time, the levels of the intermediate products (the fatty acids half-way between precursor and end product (like 20:3ω6 in the omega-6 pathway) go way down. This is a bit vexing to say the least, because if the body was cranking out lots more end products through this pathway, one would expect the levels of the intermediates to go up in the process.

The organ that is most active in this metabolism of essential fatty acids is the liver, which is hard to get samples from in humans. But in research that is currently pending publication, when we put mice on a low carb diet for a month or two and then measured the levels of $FADS_1$ and $FADS_2$ in their livers, it was reduced by 50%. But in these same animals, membrane levels of the end product fatty acids were increased and intermediates decreased, similar to what we saw in humans.

Putting this all together, along with our observation showing reduced inflammation with a low carb diet, we have to conclude that these membrane changes and reduced FADS enzyme levels indicate that much less of the end-products are getting destroyed. And although this has yet to be conclusively proven, the most likely culprit in this case of membrane vandalism is ROS (aka free radical) production that is directly linked to dietary carbohydrate intake.

Chapter 10

BODY COMPOSITION AND PHYSICAL PERFORMANCE

Introduction

When individuals embark on a program to lose weight, the implicit goal is to shed unwanted body fat. Rarely do people set out with the intended purpose to lose muscle. This seems obvious, but the importance of body composition is often overshadowed by the prompt feedback and powerful connection people have with their scale weight. There are also widespread misconceptions about the importance of dietary carbohydrate in affecting changes in body composition and exercise performance. This chapter will shed some light on these issues by providing insight into the remarkable capacity for humans to adapt to carbohydrate restriction, allowing for complete sparing of lean tissue and maintenance of physical performance in spite of significant withdrawal of carbohydrate and major cumulative weight loss.

Why Body Composition is Important

Simply put, body composition refers to the body's relative proportions or absolute contents of fat mass and lean tissue. Ideally a weight loss program will maximize fat loss and minimize muscle loss. Why? For one reason, in today's culture we tend to view too much body fat as unappealing, whereas a low body fat revealing well toned muscles is seen as being fit and attractive. Beyond aesthetic reasons, the health benefits that accompany significant weight loss are linked with reductions in body fat, not muscle. In addition, there is a growing appreciation that increased muscle mass contributes to metabolic health. More muscle translates to greater tissue volume to take up blood glucose and more mitochondria that can burn fat. That helps fend off insulin resistance and diabetes. Finally, loss of muscle will have a negative effect on physical performance and activities of daily living by decreasing strength, power, and endurance.

In reference to this last point on physical performance, it is interesting that the last three decades of national dietary guidelines espousing the health benefits of a low fat/high carbohydrate diet have occurred in parallel with the dogmatic support of sports nutritionists for carbohydrate loading. The origins of these high carbohydrate recommendations for the general population and athletes may be coincidental, but over the time they have tended to reinforce each other's position.

Weight Loss and Body Composition

How does a typical weight loss program impact fat mass and lean body mass? This depends on many variables, including (but not limited to) the level of calories and protein content, adequacy of concurrent mineral and vitamin intakes, and perhaps dietary carbohydrate content. In addition, the initial activity level and lean body mass content of the individual, plus type and amount of activity during a diet program, will be important factors in determining the net composition of the lost weight.

Most body composition assessment methods calculate the proportions of fat mass and lean body mass from estimates of body density, which are in turn derived from either assessment of body volume (density = mass/volume) or regression equations. This works because muscle is more dense (it sinks in water) whereas fat floats. So once body density is determined, it is then converted to a percent body fat (using equations developed by Siri or Brozek – see post-script), which is used to calculate fat mass and lean body mass.

These 'two-compartment models' based on body density do not address the multi-component nature of lean body mass (perhaps better called non-fat tissue), which includes other non-fat substances like water, minerals, connective tissues, and bone. In contrast, dual-energy X-ray absorptiometry (DXA) partitions out bone from the lean body mass compartment and thus provides a 3-compartment model -- fat mass soft tissue, lean body mass soft tissue, and bone (see post-script).

This direct measure of bone mineral content is clinically useful in its own right, but because bone is very dense, including it in the calculation improves the accuracy of body fat content as well. However there is another important variable that none of these techniques address. Any fluctuations in water content (e.g., reduction in extra-vascular volume or intracellular glycogen-associated water) would be interpreted as decreased lean body mass because common body composition assessment methods treat water as lean tissue. This is important in the context of carbohydrate-restricted diets because they typically reduce muscle glycogen (and its associated water) by more than half and because their natriuretic effects on the kidney can markedly reduce total body water content.

On average, a 10 kg weight loss by conventional low-fat dieting alone will result in about three-fourths of the loss from fat mass (i.e., tissue triglyceride)[74]. There are a number of reasons why this is not automatically 100%; first because adipose tissue itself is only about 85% fat, and also because energy restriction makes the body less efficient in its use of dietary protein, raising the dose needed to optimally preserve existing lean tissue. A third factor is that severely obese individuals, particularly males, accumulate extra muscle that is needed to carry the extra weight, and this is lost with the excess weight unless purposeful exercise is added to maintain muscle mass.

An even greater loss in lean body mass may be expected with weight loss approaches that contain inadequate dietary protein, minerals, or both. Combine this with a short term study that mobilizes considerable body water, and the effects of carbohydrate restriction on body composition can be conjured to appear quite negative (see Chapter 12). Therefore, it makes intuitive sense that in addition to the macronutrient makeup of the diet, both duration of a study and the diet associated mineral content could impact responses in body composition.

Dietary Macronutrient Distribution Affects Body Composition

Addressing the issue of macronutrient composition of weight loss diets on body composition responses, Krieger et al.[75] concluded from their analysis of 87 published weight loss studies that diets lower in carbohydrate were associated with greater fat loss, and also that diets providing more than the bare minimum of protein resulted in better preservation of lean body mass. These effects were independent of energy intake and participation in exercise. Translation: it's not just about eating less food. The type of macronutrients consumed has an important effect on body composition (and many other metabolic effects) too.

Very Low Carbohydrate Diets and Body Composition

Despite considerable published evidence to the contrary, there is a common belief that both muscle loss and impaired physical performance are expected to occur when individuals significantly reduce carbohydrate intake. As the logic goes, in the face of reduced carbohydrate intake, the body resorts to catabolizing protein stores for energy. Of course, as we have long since demonstrated (and discussed in Chapter 6), this is not true if an adequate period of keto-adaptation (at least 2 or more weeks) is allowed[23, 27, 76].

Let's briefly review the experimental evidence. Although results vary, on the whole studies examining body composition in response to very low carbohydrate diets do not raise any concerns about an exaggerated loss of lean tissue. In fact, properly formulated ketogenic diets have a remarkable capacity to protect muscle and exercise performance during periods of caloric restriction.

In a small but well controlled study published in 1971, Young et al.[77] examined the effects of a hypocaloric, very low carbohydrate diet on body composition and nitrogen balance in young overweight men. All foods were prepared and provided to subjects over a 9 week weight loss period. The diets each contained 1800 kcal, 115 g protein, 5 g sodium, and between 30 and 60 g carbohydrate per day. Compliance was high as evidenced by the presence of urine ketones (discussed in Chapter 13) and consistent weight loss (range 12-18 kg over 9 wk). Notably, body composition determined from underwater weighing indicated nearly all the weight loss was attributed to reductions in fat mass. There was net nitrogen (i.e., protein) loss during the first week of weight reduction but thereafter subjects were in balance or retaining nitrogen.

Over a decade later, Hoffer et al.[78] severely restricted energy intake (500 kcal/day) in overweight women for up to 8 weeks. The group who consumed a low calorie diet with adequate protein (85 g/day) plus minerals and vitamins (including sodium >5 g/day) but devoid of carbohydrate remained in positive nitrogen balance. In contrast, those subjects fed a lower protein intake (45 g protein and 45 g carbohydrate) but identical total calories were in negative protein balance. Thus even under severe caloric restriction, there is a remarkable capacity to preserve lean tissue on a low carbohydrate diet when adequate protein, vitamins, and minerals (including sodium) are provided.

Phinney et al.[27] examined metabolic adaptations to an eucaloric (i.e., energy maintenance) very low carbohydrate ketogenic diet over a 4 week period in highly trained men (bicycle racers). The diet consisted of 1.75 g/kg protein, <10 g carbohydrate, >80% of energy as fat and was supplemented with minerals including 5 g sodium. Meticulous measurements of nitrogen balance, including complete 24 hour urine and stool collections, were obtained daily. Under these conditions of constant energy and nitrogen intake, the transition from a high carbohydrate to ketogenic diet resulted in a transient loss of nitrogen during the first few days. However, the subjects then rapidly returned to positive balance by the end of the first week, where it remained for the remaining 3 weeks. Thus, over the 4 weeks of the ketogenic diet, there was an average gain of approximately 1 pound of lean body mass in highly trained subjects who continued (but did not increase) their training regimen.

This maintenance of nitrogen balance was confirmed by measurements of whole body ^{40}K counting (a direct measure of total body potassium content, which is tightly correlated with lean body mass), which showed no significant net change after the ketogenic diet. The proportion of naturally-occurring radioactive ^{40}K in human tissues is small but constant and distributes almost entirely within the intracellular compartment of fat-free mass. Thus, it provides corroborating evidence along with nitrogen balance that ketogenic diets with adequate protein and mineral intake need not result in lean tissue loss in physically active men.

Volek reported that normal-weight men who switched from their habitual diet (48% carbohydrate) to a ketogenic diet (12% carbohydrate) for 6 weeks significantly decreased fat mass (-3.4 kg) and increased lean body mass (1.1 kg)[79]. There was a significant decrease in serum insulin (-34%) and simple regression indicated that 70% of the variability in fat loss on the ketogenic diet was explained by the decrease in serum insulin concentrations. In a follow-up study in overweight men and women[80], Volek showed that a hypocaloric very low carbohydrate diet resulted in 2-fold greater whole-body fat loss than a low fat diet with a similar prescribed energy intake.

A novel and potentially clinically significant finding of this second study was that trunk fat mass comprised less of the total remaining fat mass after the low carbohydrate diet, indicating a preferential loss of fat in a region that carries a greater health risk. Specifically, this study was a crossover design, in which subjects were given both diets in randomized order, so body composition changes were determined in each subject on both diets. Fat loss in the trunk region was greater during the low carbohydrate diet in 12 of 15 men and 12 of 13 women.

In subjects with metabolic syndrome, Volek recently showed that the decrease in whole body fat mass from DXA was 1.5-fold greater after 12 weeks of a low carbohydrate than a low fat diet (5.7 kg vs 3.7 kg)[56]. The decrease in abdominal fat was 1.6-fold greater after the low carbohydrate than the low fat diet (-828 g *vs* -506 g).

The various mechanisms regulating composition of weight loss and distribution of fat loss during low carbohydrate diets remain unclear, but in large part can be attributed to factors regulating metabolic control of fuel partitioning. We have shown reliable decreases in insulin and leptin in subjects restricting carbohydrate. Insulin is the predominant hormone that inhibits lipolysis, and this effect occurs even at the lower end of its normal physiologic range. This means even small reductions in insulin may have a permissive role in fat mobilization on a low carbohydrate diet.

Importance of Resistance Training for Building Muscle

Resistance training does not affect fat loss to a great extent independent of diet. However, muscular overload induced by resistance exercise creates an anabolic stimulus for skeletal muscle fiber hypertrophy. Many studies have been conducted in the context of low fat diets and generally indicate that resistance exercise (2-3 days/week) can preserve lean body mass during weight loss. Volek and Kraemer et al.[81] showed that overweight men who consumed a low-calorie, high fiber, low fat diet and remained sedentary lost 9.6 kg of weight in 12 weeks. Two other groups consumed the same diet but added either endurance training (3 days/week working up to 50 min per session) or a combination of the same endurance training with progressive resistance training (3 days/week for 30-40 min per session). All groups showed similar weight losses. However, exercise did impact the composition of weight loss (see table). This study demonstrated on average that exercise is *not* a robust stimulus for weight loss. But the combination of dietary energy restriction with resistance training resulted in better maintenance of lean tissue during weight loss.

Body Comp (DXA)	Groups by Diet and Training Type		
	Diet	Diet + Endurance	Diet + Endurance + Resistance
Weight Loss (kg)	-9.6	-9.0	-9.9
% Loss as Fat	69	78	97
% Loss as Lean	31	22	3

Low Carbohydrate Diets and Resistance Training

Resistance training is a potent stimulus to increase muscle mass and strength, and thus there is good reason to consider weight training as an adjunct to a low carbohydrate diet for improving body composition and functional capacity. The metabolic demands of resistance exercise vary depending on the total work volume and the rest periods between sets, which can impact one's ability to tolerate different workouts on a low carbohydrate diets. Although experimental evidence is scarce, it appears most conventional types of resistance training are tolerated very well after adaptation to a low carbohydrate diet.

Jabekk et al.[82] studied untrained overweight women between 20-40 years of age, all of whom participated in a 10 week supervised resistance training program (2 workouts per week). Subjects were randomly assigned to either a hypocaloric low carbohydrate diet or to continue consuming their habitual diet. The low carbohydrate diet consisted of 23 g carbohydrate/day (6% of energy) and 95 g/day protein (22% energy). Weight loss was 5.6 kg in the low carbohydrate group, which was entirely attributed to fat loss. Thus, a low carbohydrate diet in combination with resistance training resulted in significant fat loss and complete preservation of lean body mass.

Only a few studies have directly compared diets varying in macronutrient distribution in subjects engaged in an exercise training program. Although not a very low carbohydrate diet, Layman et al.[83] reported that a moderate restriction in carbohydrate with protein intake at 1.6 g/kg (38:30:32; energy% as carb:protein:fat) resulted in more favorable body composition changes than a low fat diet with protein intake at 0.8 g/kg (61:18:26; %carb:protein:fat) in middle-aged, overweight women. All groups significantly decreased their total caloric intake by ~600 kcal/day. After 16 weeks, the moderate carbohydrate diet group with higher protein lost approximately 2.0 kg more body weight than the low fat diet group (9.3 vs. 7.3 kg). The addition of an exercise program (5 day/week walking and 2 day/week resistance training) to the moderate carbohydrate diet produced an additive effect by helping to preserve lean tissue while still allowing for better fat loss.

Volek performed a similar experiment in overweight/obese men but this time the diets were in fact low in carbohydrate and the resistance training program was more intense[84]. Men were randomized either to a low fat diet group that restricted fat to less than 25% of energy or to a very low carbohydrate ketogenic diet group that restricted carbohydrate to ~12% energy. Both groups also participated in a resistance training program (3 days/week). Body composition was assessed using DXA before and after the 12 week program. The results were compared to non-training diet only groups. As expected, the low carbohydrate diet group lost more fat, which was associated with greater decreases in insulin. Resistance training, independent of diet, resulted in increased lean body mass without compromising fat loss in both diet groups. The most dramatic reduction in percent body fat was in the low carbohydrate diet resistance training group (-5.3%), followed by low fat resistance training (-3.5%), low carbohydrate diet only (-3.4%), and low fat diet only (-2.0%) groups. These data show for the first time that resistance training is a potent stimulus to protect lean body mass in men consuming a low carbohydrate ketogenic diet while still allowing for significantly greater fat loss.

When our work is compared to the findings of Layman, a similar pattern and magnitude of change in body weight are seen across the four groups. The low carbohydrate diet groups lost more body fat, independent of training, whereas resistance training had a favorable effect on lean body mass independent of diet. The combination of a low carbohydrate diet and resistance training appears to be additive in the sense that it maximizes fat loss while preserving/increasing lean body mass and thereby results in the greatest reductions in percent body fat. Of note, none of the subjects in the ketogenic diet plus resistance training group dropped out of the study, nor did they have any problems completing the high intensity workouts. As expected with a progressive resistance training program in previously non-resistance trained subjects, they all showed marked increases in maximal strength. Thus, despite a decrease in carbohydrate availability, adaptation to a well-formulated very low carbohydrate diet allowed individuals to participate in and benefit from a high intensity strength training program.

Endurance Performance

As with resistance exercise, the dependence of endurance performance on muscle glycogen has been substantially overemphasized. Starting with the classic studies of Christensen and Hansen[85] before World War II, a string of short-term studies have been published demonstrating longer endurance exercise times with high carbohydrate diets compared to low carbohydrate diets[86]. Any study of less than 14 days duration, however, does not allow adequate time for keto-adaptation, and its results are useless in assessing the effects of a sustained low carbohydrate diet. Thus, when more recent studies using longer periods of diet adaptation to a low carbohydrate intake were done, the apparent advantages of a high carbohydrate diet were not observed[23, 76].

In these longer duration studies, when carbohydrate was kept low, with or without energy restriction, we observed no loss of peak aerobic power (VO_2max) or peak muscle strength[87]. This clearly demonstrates that dietary carbohydrate is not an obligate nutrient for the long term maintenance of muscle health and function. This observation is also consistent with the ability of a well-formulated carbohydrate restricted diet to preserve lean body mass as reported above.

Summary

As discussed elsewhere in this book, the adequate intake of minerals properly adjusted to the needs of carbohydrate restriction is essential to long term health and function. When these conditions are met, and when adequate (but not excessive) protein is provided, body mass and physical performance can be effectively maintained despite substantial restriction of dietary carbohydrate. In the clinical setting, this means that both endurance and resistance exercise are important factors that can be utilized in conjunction with carbohydrate restricted diets to optimize changes in body composition and well-being.

Post-Script: Common Body Composition Methods

BMI – Body mass index is calculated as weight in kilograms divided by height in meters squared. Values more than 25 are used as a cutoff for being overweight and more than 30 as obese. It's easy and cheap to measure, explaining why it's widely used. But BMI can overestimate body fatness in people with a lot of muscle and large frames.

UWW – Underwater weighing is based on Archimedes Principle. Body Density = Body Mass/Body Volume. If an object weighs 75 kg in air and 3 kg in water, then the loss of weight in water is equal to the weight of the volume of displaced water (i.e., 72 kg = 72 L = 72,000 cc. Density is used to calculate percent body fat (see below). UWW is considered very accurate, but it is tedious and moderately uncomfortable for the subject and limited to university laboratories. Error associated with air in lungs can be significant.

Air Plethysmography – Also known as BodPod. Fundamentally the same as underwater weighing but uses air instead of water. Measures the volume of air a person's body displaces while sitting inside a chamber rather than measuring how much water their body displaces when dunked in a tank. Same limitations as UWW.

DXA – dual-energy X-ray absorptiometry. Becoming preferred method to assess body composition. Estimates soft tissue (fat and lean) and bone mass. Uses a constant potential x-ray source to achieve a beam of dual energy radiation. X-rays passing through the body are attenuated, which is a function of tissue composition. Advantages include quick, reliable and accurate, non-invasive and minimal inconvenience, 3 compartment model, and allows regional analyses of body segments. Main disadvantages are high cost and small table dimensions. Assumes same amount of fat over bone as over neighboring bone free tissue and constant hydration and electrolyte content of lean soft tissue.

Skinfold – Based on the relationship between the fat located directly beneath the skin (subcutaneous fat) and internal fat, and body density. Calipers are used to measure the thickness of a double layer of skin and subcutaneous fat tissue. Common sites include triceps, abdominal, thigh, suprailiac, subscapular, chest, and midaxiallary. Sum of skinfolds is used in a mathematical equation to predict either body density or percent fat. Equations must be population specific *(i.e., similar age, gender, state of training, fatness, race)* in order to be accurate. Accuracy is also highly dependent on the skill of the person performing the test.

Computing Percent Body Fat (Siri Equation): % Fat = (495/Density) – 450

Assumes density Fat Tissue = 0.90 g/cc and density Lean Tissue = 1.10 g/cc

Assumptions: Densities of fat and lean tissues remain constant even with large individual variations in total body fat; lean tissue components of bone and muscle are essentially the same density among different individuals, but this has been questioned in certain ethnic groups, growing children, and aging adults. Based upon the chemical analysis of a small number of human corpses, none of whom were obese[88].

Chapter 11

PERSONALIZED NUTRITION

Introduction

When we are introduced to people as 'nutritionists', we're inevitably asked... *what should I eat?* Our usual answer...*it depends.* And if the conversation continues and we get around to telling them our research is focused on very low carbohydrate diets, the question almost always pops up...*how much should I restrict my carbohydrate?* Again, our answer... *it depends?* These answers are certainly concise, and also scientifically true, but they really beg the logical follow up question...*depends on what?* That's where the conversation starts to get complicated, but also really fascinating, because it cuts right to the heart of personalized nutrition.

The last few years have brought incredible progress in genetics, particularly to methods for measuring DNA and clinical biomarkers. Along with these scientific and analytical advancements has come the promise of personalized approaches to lifestyle. The recognition that two individuals respond differently to the same diet and therefore require unique combinations of nutrients for optimal health is oddly juxtaposed with long-standing national dietary guidelines that promote a one size fits all approach. Along these lines, papers encouraging dietitians to study genetics in preparation for personalized nutrition are published simultaneously with ones condemning any diet outside narrow guidelines. We're optimistic that this dichotomy between hedging for the future of personalized nutrition coupled with an unwillingness to break from tradition is temporary, although we dare not define temporary.

Despite some reluctance on the part of many dietitians, doctors, and policy makers to break from cookie cutter diet treatments, many entrepreneurs are attempting to capitalize on the promise of personalized nutrition. There is no shortage of companies that will gladly accept a small cheek swab with a fair amount of cash and in return provide you a customized diet and supplement plan. Are the results based on scientific research? And more important, are they helpful? The truth is it's hard to tell. We're far from having precisely defined genetic testing for personal diet prescription. The prudent advice for now is to have a healthy dose of skepticism.

The aim of this chapter is to provide some technical background and frame some of the relevant issues and challenges that need to be addressed in moving toward a more personalized approach to diet, especially as it pertains to carbohydrate intake. In this regard, there may be some novel signs that can be used to dial in on your level of carbohydrate tolerance.

Diet and Variability

We readily accept the idea that people differ in appearance, intellect, physical performance, preferences for music, art, sports, and of course food. Therefore, the need to customize diets should come as no surprise. But what is the evidence? Some of the best proof showing the genetic contribution to the variability in weight loss comes from studies in monozygotic 'genetically identical' twins. Drs. Claude Bouchard and Angelo Tremblay conducted two such experiments in the 1990s that examined the variability in changes in body weight in response to negative and positive energy balance in relation to genetics[89].

In the positive energy balance experiment, twins were overfed 1000 kcal/day (6 days out of 7) for 100 days. There was a wide discrepancy in weight gain ranging from about 9 to 30 pounds between the different pairs of twins, but weight gain within each twin pair was quite similar. Specifically, the between twin variance in weight gain was three times the variance within pairs. When looking at gains in upper body fat or abdominal visceral fat, the between twin variance was six times greater than within pairs.

In the negative energy balance experiment, twins exercised twice a day (9 days out of 10) for 93 days, while each individual's dietary energy intake was held at their sedentary maintenance energy level. This created a daily deficit of 624 kcal/day for everyone in the study. Similar to the weight gain findings, there was a surprisingly wide discrepancy in weight loss among the different pairs of twin ranging from 2 to 18 pounds, while weight loss within twins was again very similar. These well controlled prospective twin studies demonstrate a remarkable level of variability in weight and fat loss between twin pairs. In contrast, the much smaller variance in changes in weight, especially fat mass, within twins provides convincing evidence for the role of genetic factors in determining how our bodies respond to both energy deficit and energy surplus.

A role for genetics in other biologic responses can be inferred from well controlled studies where the same nutrient composition is fed to subjects. In a recent very low carbohydrate feeding experiment in men we observed a wide range of responses in some variables (e.g., LDL-C), whereas other variables showed a considerably lower variance (e.g., triglycerides, HDL-C). For example the average LDL-C response was +6 mg/dL, but when looking at individual responses one subject increased 53 mg/dL whereas another decreased 41 mg/dL despite consuming the same diet[30]! What this means is that genes have a major role in how you respond to diet and exercise. It is possible, for example, that if you exercise vigorously you may see very little benefit in terms of weight loss, but you may be programmed to be responsive to other stimuli like carbohydrate restriction.

Nutrigenetics and Nutrigenomics

Two recently coined terms that come up when studying the interplay between diet and genes are 'nutrigenetics' and 'nutrigenomics'. They are intimately related, at times overlapping, concepts that share a common goal of elucidating the way diet and genes interact to impact susceptibility to disease. Both are directed at understanding how genetic variation explains differences in the dietary responses of individuals. For example, suppose that you and your co-worker agree to eat the exact same diet for one month. Results of laboratory work indicate your co-worker's cholesterol increased while yours decreased. A nutrigenetic approach would look at just a few gene candidates ('suspects') and aim to determine the genetic differences between you and your co-worker and how those genetic variations (alleles) relate to your distinct cholesterol responses.

Nutrigenomics, on the other hand is concerned with discovery... it looks at many genes at once. A nutrigenomics approach might involve extracting a small piece of adipose tissue from you and your co-worker before and after your 1-month diet to measure the activity of an array of hundreds of genes to see which ones were responsive to the diet. Sometimes the gene products (proteins, metabolites) are measured, so nutrigenomics is tightly linked with 'proteomics' and 'metabolomics'. In short nutrigenetics analyzes how genetic variation among people allows them to respond differently to the same diet or the same supplement, whereas nutrigenomics refers to how nutrients alter gene expression. Sometimes distinguishing between the two is not clear-cut and some experts prefer to use a catch all term like *nutritional genomics* to describe any effort that probes the relationships between genes and diet.

Complexity of Nutritional Signals

Nutrients are broadly classified into 4 macronutrient categories (carbohydrate, fat, protein, alcohol) that provide energy. We also need a regular source of several essential micronutrients (vitamins, minerals) that our body cannot make and we therefore must obtain from food. There are also a host of other nonessential chemicals in food broadly referred to as phytonutrients that can elicit important effects on metabolism and health. Therefore when we eat typical meals consisting of multiple foods, the body must process potentially a hundred or more different chemical signals.

These nutrient signals in turn induce robust hormonal responses that further impact regulatory control over a broad range of physiologic processes, and these responses can differ greatly depending on both the macronutrient and micronutrient compositions of the diet. Moreover, there are important interactive effects that change the way the body processes nutrients. For example, iron is handled very differently by the body when consumed with vitamin C, and saturated fat intake has a variable effect in the body depending on how much carbohydrate is consumed along with it. And finally, when you add other variables like dosage and timing of ingestion that can also change the signal dynamics, the vast permutations of nutrient signals impacting physiologic outcomes become an extraordinarily complex system to study.

Complexity of the Genome

The genome consists of over 3 billion base pairs made up of long chains of adenine, guanine, cytosine and thymine on the 23 chromosomes. Humans have about 21,000 genes, each encoding a protein, scattered around the genome. The length of DNA that contains a typical gene extends about 50,000 base pairs, of which only a fraction, say 1,000—actually encode the protein sequence. This means the majority of the genome (~98%) consists of expanses of DNA whose function(s) remain unknown. This is sometimes called 'junk' DNA. Interestingly, functions are being found for some of this junk. For example some noncoding DNA sequences are genetic "switches" that regulate when and where genes are expressed. One expert estimates that 5% of the non-coding DNA has a function. So whether a DNA variant is found in a gene or in a non-coding expanse of DNA, it may have meaning for some yet unknown dietary response.

Any one person's DNA is about 99-99.5% identical to any other person's DNA. There are two major causes of person-to-person genetic differences. The major cause is named copy number variants. These are many different places in the DNA where the number of copies of a gene can vary from one to many hundreds. For instance, on average, people from cultures that historically have high starch diets (such as Japanese and European Americans) have more copies of the gene salivary amylase than people from cultures that historically eat low starch diets (such as Mbuti and Yakut)[90]. Amylase is involved in digesting carbohydrates. More copies of the salivary amylase gene is correlated with more enzymatic activity. Many but not all genes exhibit copy number variation in humans. Some of these copy variants show evidence of adaptations that took place over a million years ago, while others show evidence for selection by diet only in the last few thousand years.

The second most abundant source of person-to-person variation in DNA consists of single nucleotide polymorphisms (SNPs). A SNP is a place in the DNA where one of the four nucleotides has been replaced by another. These SNPs may change the function or amount of any of our 21,000 proteins. So far, scientists have identified about 20 million SNPs but many more exist. Overall any two people differ for about 3 million SNPs, which is about 0.1% of their total DNA. As an example, SNPs in the Lactase gene are responsible for the persistence of Lactase expression in adults which allows for adults to drink milk – lactose tolerance. Most cultures that kept milk producing animals, such as cows, camels, and goats independently evolved different SNPs in the Lactase gene that allow for lactose tolerance. The task of finding which SNPs and copy number variants are important in respect to nutritional genomics will certainly be challenging. Although the effects of a 0.5-1% difference may seem small, the overall effects on physiology can be large. For example some of the polymorphisms in genes that code for enzymes involved in carbohydrate digestion (i.e., amylase and lactase) are the result of selection acting on human populations eating varying amounts of starch and lactose.

Personalized Nutrition – Where to Start?

It seems reasonable to target nutrients that represent dietary triggers capable of pushing someone from susceptibility to disease. Since they are consumed in larger quantities, it makes sense that macronutrients would exert some of the most powerful signals.

Why We Respond More Acutely to Carbohydrate than to Fat Intake

Depending on dose and timing of dietary carbohydrate, blood glucose can exhibit large and rapid excursions. However failure to maintain an adequate supply of glucose can have dire consequences; thus our bodies ardently defended a minimum blood glucose level. Falling below this minimum (in the absence of blood ketones) triggers prompt physiological responses to maintain glucose levels necessary for brain. In contradistinction, blood fat levels (either as triglycerides or free fatty acids) are neither sensed nor monitored to the same degree or in the same way as glucose. The need to sense fatty acid levels is not as vital for minute-to-minute functioning.

There are a number of reasons why defining an individualized carbohydrate level is a logical target. First, the potential range of human dietary carbohydrate intake is remarkably broad. At one extreme, because it is not actually essential in the human diet, intake can be very low. At the other extreme, most healthy humans can tolerate carbs in relatively large quantities for extended periods without toxicity. Thus, there is a wide range of intakes that can be compatible with health. Second, the consumption of carbohydrates trigger potent downstream regulatory elements that induce a unique metabolic state orchestrated through several key transcription factors.

Human Adaptability and Carbohydrate

As humans we share a common physiology in the way cells, tissues, organs and systems are put together and respond to stimuli. Along these lines one of the most impressive aspects of human physiology is the ability to adapt to varying nutritional input. Take an average person habitually consuming over half her/his calories from carbohydrate and then abruptly deprive that person of this nutrient. Perhaps 'that person' is you. Over the course of a week or two you will observe a robust and coordinated set of adaptations go into motion that results in nearly perfect metabolic control. This adaptability to a changing dietary input is one of the marvels of the human body, but this variability is also one of the least appreciated aspects of nutritional science. Not everyone has the same 'skill' in adapting to dietary change.

Does everyone respond to *reducing* dietary carbohydrate in a uniform manner? In other words is there variability in the way people respond to removing the majority of carbohydrate from their diet? While the time required for adaptation may vary, and it certainly takes at least 2 weeks, the end result of this adaptation is the same. Starvation experiments or studies that severely restricted dietary carbohydrate indicate a consistent shift in metabolic fuel partitioning with little variability. Typically, nobody dies or even loses consciousness. You could interpret that to mean we are hardwired to respond to carbohydrate restriction in a reliable and 'healthy' manner.

But what if we ask the corollary question; does everyone respond to *increasing* carbohydrate in a consistent manner? In this case, the results are likely not as predictable. Some people can tolerate moderate to high levels of carbohydrate without signs or symptoms of metabolic distress. However, others will struggle to maintain health (e.g., normal blood glucose and lipids) under an increasing 'carbohydrate challenge'. From a genetic perspective, this means the ability to thrive under a low carbohydrate diet is highly conserved, whereas the ability to tolerate a higher carbohydrate intake is less so.

What does this tell us in terms of personalized nutrition? One could take the position that a low carbohydrate intake is the 'normal' metabolic state associated with health. This is consistent with the view that the majority of human evolution occurred in the backdrop of a low carbohydrate intake. The ability to tolerate more dietary carbohydrate is clearly a problem for many. Consider the recent uncontrolled experiment in which approximately 200 million adults in the United States have been encouraged to consume higher levels of dietary carbohydrate in place of fat. In the same time frame, more than half of us have ended up overweight or obese. The results from this national level experience point us to the logical conclusion that the ability to remain healthy with increasing levels of carbohydrate is limited to a subset of the population. Therefore determining who those people are and what characteristics give them the ability to consume carbohydrate without untoward effects is a major question that can and should be addressed.

We have already explained that insulin resistance, metabolic syndrome, and type 2 diabetes are all manifestations of carbohydrate intolerance. In other words, if you have one of these conditions you are sensitive (in a negative context) to the effects of carbohydrate. To what extent this is a reflection of genetic variation remains unclear. However, in our opinion, finding an objective means to define the optimal carbohydrate intake for an individual represents 'low hanging fruit' in our quest to develop nutritional genomics and personalized nutrition.

How Much Does Genotype Matter?

How much of the variability in a given phenotype like body weight or body mass index is attributed to genotype? Although there is some debate depending on the specific study and methodological approach, genetics probably accounts for 50-80% of the variability in BMI. The hard truth is that finding the specific genes responsible has been a disappointment. The contribution of any given individual SNP variant to weight loss is relatively small. When multiple SNPs are combined, it is possible to harness the information and explain the total genetic contribution to the variability in diet response. Complex diseases like type 2 diabetes are not due to a single gene, they are polygenetic (i.e., diseases that depend on the simultaneous presence of several genes). Studies that have measured millions of genes in large cohorts have discovered a total of 38 SNPs associated with type 2 diabetes[91]. These genetic variants only explain about 10% of type 2 diabetes heritability meaning there still remain several we have not yet discovered. It is likely that all the known SNPs will need to be included and statistically manipulated to begin to account for the total contribution of genetics and develop useful tools for clinical prediction. This has not been done yet in large numbers of subjects eating widely different carbohydrate intakes or any diet for that matter.

Personalizing Diet, Beyond Genetics

When considering the reasons for variability in response to diet, undoubtedly genetics plays a role, but can you personalize your diet with non-genetic markers? As discussed in Chapter 7, a randomized clinical trial (the 'A to Z Study') comparing weight loss responses to diets low and high in carbohydrate indicated that the level of insulin resistance was an important determinant of success. In the initial publication[43], after one year women assigned the low carbohydrate diet lost more than twice the weight (10.6 lbs) than women assigned the high carbohydrate diet (4.8 lbs). These data are consistent with multiple recent studies comparing high carbohydrate to low carbohydrate diets for weight loss.

However in a follow up analysis of the original study data (which has been published only in abstract form)[44], when women assigned to the high carbohydrate and low carbohydrate groups were divided into tertiles based on baseline insulin levels as a marker of insulin resistance, the results were striking. In the low carbohydrate diet group, weight loss was similar in the most insulin sensitive (11.7 lbs) and insulin resistant (11.9 lbs) tertiles. However weight loss with the high carbohydrate diet was significantly greater in the insulin sensitive (9.0 lbs) than in the insulin resistant (3.3 lbs) tertiles. Thus insulin-sensitive women experienced a similar success independent of which diet they were assigned, but the more insulin resistant women fared poorly when assigned a diet high in carbohydrate compared to a low carbohydrate diet.

This is consistent with the concept that insulin resistance is a manifestation of carbohydrate intolerance, and demonstrates this condition is best treated with a diet that limits carbohydrate. Moreover, this is the first human study to demonstrate that a clinical biomarker (insulin resistance) can be used to segregate weight loss responses to a specific diet. While this segregation of individuals towards a diet that will best suit them for weight loss is helpful, it does not inform those individuals if and how much to restrict carbohydrate to optimize chances for long-term weight maintenance.

Markers of Carbohydrate Intolerance Beyond Insulin

If you have carbohydrate intolerance, metabolically this translates to a propensity to divert dietary carbohydrate away from skeletal muscle and towards the liver. And if liver glycogen stores are full, a significant portion of your additional dietary carbohydrates will be converted to fat. Outside of elevated serum triglycerides and an increase in liver triglyceride content (steatosis), a person cannot see, feel or otherwise detect this stealth-like conversion of carbohydrate to fat until a lot of damage has been done. It would be helpful to identify an early signal of this insidious diversion of carbohydrate into fat.

In this case, genetic analysis is not yet possible because not enough is known. When and if genetics can be used to predict propensity to convert carbohydrates into fat is unknown. If you are consuming too many carbohydrates, it is helpful to have an objective measure on how your body is handling the digested sugar for long-term success. Over the long term, exceeding your carbohydrate tolerance is associated with slowed weight loss or even weight gain, so you might use the scale or perhaps various body circumference measures (e.g., waist, hip). Failure to see downward trends in these measures is a sign you have exceeded your level of carbohydrate tolerance.

However, it can take weeks or even months to accurately detect lack of progress. That's a lot of valuable time wasted. If you obtained blood work, certain clinical markers will increase when too many carbohydrates are being ingested. Most notable will be an increase in triglycerides. While this can serve as a reasonable gauge as to whether you have exceeded your carbohydrate limit, values do vary from day to day and there is the expense and inconvenience of having to have your blood drawn and analyzed on a repeated basis.

Serum Triglyceride Level vs Composition

Triglyceride levels in plasma are a function of how fast they are entering the bloodstream compared to how quickly they are being removed. After any previous meal has been digested and absorbed, the only source of new triglyceride in the circulation is the liver, which secretes VLDL made from free fatty acids, other lipoprotein remnants, or fatty acids newly made from glucose (i.e., lipogenesis). Given this complex balance of factors, it would be very desirable to have a specific biomarker of newly made fat to quantitate the degree on ongoing lipogenesis.

As discussed in Chapter 9, palmitoleic acid (POA) can effectively serve this role, as its only significant dietary sources are macadamia nuts and avocados. This potential biomarker of carbohydrate intolerance has the advantage over SNPs in that POA changes in response to one's diet. Thus it has the capability to assist the individual in finding the correct level of dietary carbohydrate intake to avoid substantial conversion of carbohydrate to fat, and thus tailor one's diet to that level of carbohydrate than can be efficiently metabolized. An obvious advantage of measuring POA is that its production by the liver is determined by the downstream sum of many factors that determine inter-organ glucose exchange. Thus it is one measure influenced by many physiologic and genetic inputs, giving it an advantage over measuring a few SNPs in this overall pathway and trying to assess their combined effect.

Summary

There is a strong biologically based argument for tailoring diets to individuals. Effects of different types and amounts of food on health and weight vary widely between individuals. Although these general observations reflect reproducible peer reviewed science, specific recommendations for individuals based on DNA analysis are not ready for prime time – despite the commercial availability of nutrigenomic analyses.

Developing the tools for DNA based nutritional recommendations is a very active area of research. The challenge is to demystify the process and unravel the intricacies of how people respond to food so that knowledge can be translated into routine clinical management of patient care. Over the next decade, personalized nutrition can be expected to hit the nutrition field like a tsunami – best to be ahead of the wave.

Chapter 12

LOW CARBOHYDRATE RESEARCH PITFALLS

Introduction

When a research paper is published in a peer-reviewed journal, we are conditioned to think of it as an observation that probably can be believed as true until it is either confirmed or refuted by subsequent research. You observe something new and report it. Your observation is subjected to scrutiny and it either holds up or not. If it does, you get credit for the discovery. This is plain vanilla science.

But in the real world, when a research paper is published that reinforces a concept that we very much want to believe, 'we' – the mainstream consensus – treat it as dogma. After all, if we want to believe that a few thousand years of agricultural exposure has irrevocably shifted our genetic makeup away from a couple of million years of evolutionary pressure generated by our hunting ancestors, what's to stop us?

If this sounds overly cynical to you the reader, please accept our apologies. But if you have ever tried to argue the case for data over dogma, perhaps this sounds familiar.

But let's frame it another way. Every year or so, there's a high profile case in which a scientist fabricates data to generate a high profile publication. This is clear scientific malfeasance. Fame, fortune, and federal grants ride on high profile publications. Some of these people forfeit their research careers, and some go to jail.

But what rarely makes the news is the much more common situation where a scientist designs a study with a particular result in mind. Say that your preliminary data tell you that you'll probably see the result you want after 1 week or 2 weeks, but that result wouldn't be likely to persist if you continue for 4 or 6 weeks. Is it wrong to do just a 2 week study?

Another surprisingly common situation is that a scientist chooses not to publish 'embarrassing data', or decides to present it in a way that avoids the reader drawing the logical (but embarrassing) conclusion. But isn't there a peer-review 'checks and balances' system in place to ensure proper scientific methods and that logical conclusions are made? Yes, ideally this is true, but the reality is that the peer-review system is far from perfect, and in particular tends to favor findings in line with the consensus. More often than not, editors and anonymous experts chosen to review the paper give their uncritical acceptance rather than grapple with the uncomfortable data. On occasion an astute reviewer may call-out the scientist with the comment "your data do not support your conclusions", but this is more of a rarity than the norm.

What would motivate a scientist to take a chance that s/he might get such feedback.

Can we all say 'peer-pressure'? How about 'calculated risk'?

What We Publish, And What We Cite

Science, in general, and the nutritional sciences in particular, have become highly conformist. Smart scientists go to their scientific meetings, listen to the discussion, and come to understand what is acceptable and what is not. Those who ignore this readily available information do so at their own risk. Non-conformists tend to have trouble getting papers published and research grants funded.

The second level of control over the 'impact' of what is published is the number of times a peer-reviewed publication is cited in subsequent published papers. If your paper gets cited by another scientist, it's usually a sign of acceptance or esteem. If you want your career to advance, you need your peers to cite your published papers. The more 'impact' (i.e., citations) your papers have, the better your reputation as a scientist. And citations are a very subjective behavior. If your peers like your paper's conclusions, it will get cited much more than if your conclusions force them to change their perspective on a topic.

Here are three classic examples from the low carbohydrate diet literature.

The Yang and Van Itallie Study

In 1976, Dr. Theodore Van Itallie (yes, the same one who accused Dr. Atkins of "gross inaccuracies" in 1973[16]) and his junior colleague from Columbia University published a paper in the highly respected Journal of Clinical Investigation. It was entitled "Composition of weight lost during short term weight reduction"[92]. Drs. Yang and Van Itallie gave extremely obese male subjects either a relatively low protein (50 g/d) diet containing 90 g/d of carbohydrate, or the same protein with low carb (10 g/d) for 10 days each in a crossover study. The fat contents of these two liquid diets were adjusted so that both diets delivered 800 Calories per day, and the sodium (1.3 g/d) and potassium contents (2.4 g/d) were also identical across the two diets. Using the best techniques of the time, the investigators measured total weight loss and the composition of that weight loss across each 10-day period.

The reported rates of weight loss for the subjects were: high carb diet 0.28 kg per day, low carb 0.47 kg per day. The rates of nitrogen (i.e., lean tissue) loss were: high carb diet 1.6 g/d, low carb diet 2.9 g/d. These two rates of lean tissue loss did not differ significantly, and since a gram of nitrogen is the amount in an ounce of lean tissue, even the cumulative difference over 10 days (i.e., less than a pound of lean tissue) was not physiologically significant. Fat losses during the two diet periods were similar (not surprising as dietary energy intakes were identical), and thus the differences in weight loss were due to much greater loss of water during the low carbohydrate diet.

In their discussion, the authors noted that the more rapid weight loss with the low carbohydrate diet was due to water loss, accounting for 61% of the total. They also commented on the "slightly greater" loss of lean tissue during the low carbohydrate diet, even though this was not a statistically significant difference between the two diets (and thus scientifically inaccurate). Interestingly, the authors ended their discussion with the acknowledgement that data from a short-term study such as theirs might not predict the human response to a longer period of carbohydrate and energy restriction.

As of this writing, this paper has been cited 116 times in the peer-reviewed literature. The most common reason for its being cited is to emphasize (incorrectly) that most of the weight loss with a low carbohydrate diet is due to water loss, while others make reference to the greater (sic) rate of lean tissue loss. And in general discussion about low carbohydrate diets, this flawed conclusion is famously offered as proof of the futility of carbohydrate restriction.

Now, for comparison, let's contrast the response to this study with that to another similar study published 8 years later in 1984. Entitled 'Metabolic effects of very low calorie weight reduction diets', this study was done by Dr. Hoffer and colleagues at MIT and Harvard, and was also published in the Journal of Clinical Investigation[78]. So, similarly prestigious institutions and the same excellent journal. However Dr. Hoffer's paper has only been cited 77 times – one third less often than the Van Itallie study. Why might this be?

Perhaps it is because Dr. Hoffer studied moderately overweight women given low and high carbohydrate diets of about 700 Calories per day for 6-8 weeks and found <u>no difference in their rates of weight loss</u>. But provocatively, what he also found was that his low carbohydrate diet (providing a more effective protein level for dieting subjects – 1.5 g/kg reference weight per day) resulted in significantly <u>better</u> preservation of lean tissue and physical performance compared to the same number of calories as a mixture of protein (0.8 g/kg – the current DRI) plus carbohydrate.

In essence, what Dr. Hoffer's study demonstrated was that in the context of energy restriction, protein is more effective at preserving lean body mass than an equal number of calories as carbohydrate. But this was not what the mainstream nutrition consensus wanted to hear, so most of the 'experts' tried to ignore this well-controlled study done under conditions much more relevant to the real world of weight loss diets than Van Itallie's short-term study of his low protein, high fat diet.

There were other very important lessons to be gleaned from Dr. Hoffer's study. At the time of both his and Dr. Van Itallie's studies, it had been known for decades that both total starvation and severe carbohydrate restriction increase excretion of sodium by the kidneys. Known technically as 'the natriuresis of fasting', there was active research being done in that period to elucidate the physiological mechanism of this phenomenon. In Dr. Van Itallie's study, he gave his subjects 1.3 g/d of sodium, and those on the low carb diet lost a lot of body water (presumably due to the natriuresis effect). It is also very likely that they were constantly light-headed, dizzy, and easily fatigued given this combination of a low carbohydrate diet and a very low sodium intake. In contrast, Dr. Hoffer's subjects were given 5 grams of sodium per day, and there was: a) no difference in water weight loss between his two diet groups, and b) his low carb subjects had no headache, no dizziness, and their endurance performance (assessed in a separate concurrent study) was as good or better than the subjects given the mixed diet.

Now, you might ask, isn't it tantamount to subject abuse to give them 5 grams of sodium per day? Wasn't that harmful? The simple answer is, no. The reason: all carbohydrate-restricted diets, even ones providing 50-60 grams of carbohydrate like Dr. Hoffer's mixed diet, are natriuretic – they make the kidneys dump sodium. Now, if you are bloated, edematous, or hypertensive, 'dumping sodium' is a good thing. But if you do not (or no longer) have these fluid-excess symptoms, then over-excretion of sodium results in the above list of symptoms. And more worrisome, it can have negative health effects as well.

Sodium is the positively charged ion that the body uses in its circulating fluid (serum and extracellular fluid) to balance the concentration of positive charges from potassium that is concentrated inside cells. The membrane enzyme sodium-potassium ATPase is the ion pump that keeps both of these cations separated and in the right place. For nerves, muscles, and other cellular functions to work right, neither of these ion concentrations can deviate much from that of the other. With severe sodium restriction (like 1.3 grams per day, combined with the natriuretic effects of carbohydrate restriction), the body responds first by mobilizing any excess extracellular fluid (which is why bloating disappears) and then by contracting its circulating volume. It is this contracted circulating volume that causes dizziness, headache, and ease of fatigue.

At some point, when confronted with this low sodium intake plus carbohydrate restriction, most people's defense mechanisms can't maintain normal mineral balances. So the body's next level of defense is for the adrenal gland to secrete the hormone aldosterone, which makes kidney tubular cells excrete potassium in order to conserve sodium. That is, the body wastes some of its intracellular potassium in order to cling to whatever sodium it can. However unless there is copious potassium coming in from the diet, this excess urinary potassium comes from the body's potassium pool inside cells. Two things then happen. First, nerve and muscle cells don't work well, leading to cardiac dysrhythmias and muscle cramps. Second, because potassium is an obligate component of lean tissue, the body starts losing muscle even if there's plenty of protein in the diet.

Clearly none of these effects of sodium restriction are desirable, particularly when one is trying to lose body fat while retaining as much lean tissue as possible. Luckily, if in the context of a low carbohydrate diet you give the subject/patient a total of 5 grams of sodium per day (for example 2-3 grams on their food and 2 grams as broth/bouillon), none of these bad things happen. And what about blood pressure? Typically, during a diet providing less than 50 grams of carbohydrate and 5 grams per day of sodium, blood pressure stays in the low normal range, even in formerly hypertensive subjects just recently off their anti-hypertensive medication.

So, were there any negative side effects of Van Itallie's low carb, low sodium diet on his research subjects? Luckily, apparently nothing major, but the 10-day study period was short enough that major cumulative effects were unlikely. Thus its primary negative effect was to give fuel to critics of low carbohydrate diets, some of whom to this day still claim that this study shows that most of the weight lost on a low carbohydrate diet is water. And this view persists in spite of the many subsequent longer-term studies (like Dr. Hoffer's with adequate sodium, potassium, and protein) that demonstrate that even without added resistance training, from 70-90% of one's weight loss comes from adipose triglyceride.

The Yale Turkey Study

This is an amazing (and completely true) tale.

In 1980, the prestigious New England Journal of Medicine published a study by Dr. Felig's group at Yale, in which they compared a 400 Calorie "protein diet" to a 400 Calorie diet consisting of half protein and half carbohydrate[93]. The protein source used in both diets was boiled turkey, the carbohydrate source was grape juice, and the diet durations varied from 3-5 weeks. Across the duration of the diets, whole body protein losses were modest and not significantly different, but the subjects on the protein diet lost a lot more sodium while appearing to gain a substantial amount of potassium. They also reported low blood pressure in the protein diet subjects, along with reduced plasma norepinephrine levels. The authors concluded that the protein (i.e., low carbohydrate) diet interfered with the adrenergic nervous system and normal blood pressure control. This indictment of low carbohydrate diets has been cited 145 times in the peer-reviewed literature.

Within a few days of its publication, a number of letters were submitted to the journal protesting the methods used by the authors of this study. But although the paper was published in February, the letters were not published until 5 months later. In their responses to these letters, the original authors were allowed by the editor (a personal friend of Dr. Felig, and the latter also served on the Journal's editorial board) to discount the stated concerns without actually answering them.

So, what was so bad about this paper? Well, first there was the problem of giving a very low carbohydrate diet, known to elicit the 'natriuresis of fasting' without giving enough sodium to prevent overt and dangerous symptoms. The authors claimed that they held sodium intake low and constant across the two diets in order to be able to precisely measure the balance of intake versus output.

Second (and most fascinating), although they had a number of experienced research physicians on their team, they made an obvious procedural error in performing the study. As noted above, for their sole dietary protein they used 'boiled turkey', which they chose because they wanted to have a uniform source of protein so they could precisely measure each subject's daily intake. This, when balanced against urinary nitrogen excretion (the primary measure of protein breakdown), allowed them to determine if the subjects had a net retention or loss of protein.

But here was their problem. Rather than measure how much protein was in the boiled turkey, they used the protein (and potassium) values for raw turkey from a standard handbook of food composition. Their rationale for doing this was that they only boiled slices of turkey breast for about 30 minutes to soften them, so assumed that losses of protein and potassium into the broth were negligible.

For an experienced nutritionist, however, it was obvious from the data published in their paper that such losses were not negligible. Why? Because in whole-body balance studies like this one lasting for a period of weeks, when the body loses nitrogen, it also loses potassium. This is because lean tissue contains a lot of potassium, so changes in one are usually highly correlated with changes in the other. This is one of the basic tenants of mammalian metabolism. But in Dr. Felig's subjects on the protein diet, they appeared to average about 2 ounces of lean tissue loss per day, but 'gained' a lot of potassium over the same period. Because potassium and nitrogen contents of the body generally track together, this should have been a huge red flag for both the authors and the reviewers of this paper, but it was ignored by both. This paper got published and has been cited over a hundred times, despite having a huge methodological flaw and drawing the wrong conclusions.

Here's what happened, and how we figured it out within a couple of days of its publication. Aboriginal hunters (or more likely their wives and mothers-in-law) have known from time immemorial that if you boil meat, you must drink the broth to stay well. But back in the winter of 1980, we had to re-invent this wheel. Simple physiology dictates that when an animal is killed, within less than a minute, ATP in the muscles is depleted and sodium-potassium ATPase ceases to function. That means that by the time any meat reaches a cooking pot, lots of the intra-cellular potassium has leaked through membranes and equilibrated with the fluid outside of cells. So when meat is boiled, particularly if it is sliced into half-inch thick slices, lots of the potassium it contains leaks out into the broth.

To confirm this, we took fresh turkey breast, sliced it one-half inch thick, and boiled it in distilled water (one pound of meat in a quart of water) for exactly 30 minutes. Then we (by which I mean Marie Marcucci, the head technician in the GCRC Lab at MIT) analyzed the broth for potassium, comparing this result to the handbook value for potassium in turkey breast. What we found was that 45% of the potassium in the meat came out into the broth. This means that if you want to consume all of the potassium that was in the meat, you'd have to drink the broth. The Osage did it, the Inuit did it, but these Yale scientists didn't. Or more precisely, they didn't have their research subjects do it.

So how does this explain the anomaly in this study's results? Let's use a simple financial analogy. You do something that earns you $100. Every day you do it, and after 30 days you assume you've earned $3000. But you forget that you have to pay 45% tax on your income (done by automatic monthly deductions from your account). Meanwhile, every day you spend $60 for housing, food, and whatever. At the end of the month, you think you have $1200 left, but when you check your bank account, you discover you are $150 in the hole!

153

So in effect the Yale scientists credited each subject with 100 mEq of potassium intake when they only got 55. If their urine contained 70 mEq, they assumed that the other 30 mEq were retained, and that's what they reported. But in reality, with 70 mEq coming out for every 55 going in, each subject was losing 15 mEq of potassium from body stores, driven by aldosterone because they were being sodium restricted. And because having adequate potassium in muscle is an obligate requirement to maintain muscle protein synthesis, this potassium deficit drove muscle protein breakdown despite an apparently adequate dietary protein intake.

That was 1980. They published a study with a blatant methodological error that distorted their results, we pointed it out, but they were allowed to skate. So what harm was done, and why make such a big deal out of it 30 years later? The short answer is that a study was done by a group with known hostility to low carbohydrate diets (e.g., see Dr. Felig's hostile editorials in NEJM in 1978[94] and 1984[95]). They got the answer that they wanted (but not supported by their data), and the untruth that it promoted persists today.

And why dredge all this old history up now?

If we can't recognize our past errors, how do we progress?

Carbohydrate Loading

A beloved mainstay of sports nutrition is the concept that a high carbohydrate intake is required to support high intensity performance. And the equally fondly held corollary of this is that low carbohydrate diets impair one's capacity for exercise. And of course, there are copious studies that support these views.

The classic study leading to the practice of carbohydrate loading was done by two Danish scientists, Christensen and Hansen, and published in 1939[85]. They gave trained athletes one of three diets, mixed, high fat, or high carbohydrate for periods of 7 days each before having them ride to exhaustion on a stationary bicycle. Their observation was pretty straight-forward: the more carbohydrate in the diet, the longer the subject could pedal.

This concept was picked up in the 1960s by a team of Swedish scientists[86], one of whom (Dr. Jonas Bergstrom) had developed a needle that allowed muscle biopsies to be obtained without surgery. Using this needle, they were able to show a direct correlation between the amount of glycogen in a muscle and the duration of exercise that muscle could sustain. Their data were clear and unequivocal, and many similar studies done by others have confirmed their findings.

But there is just one minor issue with this whole body of research; in a word, duration. Christensen and Hansen used 7 day diets, Bergstrom's group used 7-10 days, and many others used periods of diet adaptation as short as 4 days. When a Swedish colleague of this group was asked why they didn't use longer periods of adaptation to the low carbohydrate, high fat diet, he replied that they couldn't get athletes to eat that much protein for any longer period. It seems that their idea of a low carbohydrate diet was to feed their subjects lots of lean steak!

This is an interesting twist, given the long and successful history of Scandinavian explorers in the Arctic. In 1885-6, Nansen and Johansen left the research ship Fram and made an attempt at reaching the North Pole[96]. On their return, they came ashore on an uninhabited island north of Russia where they were stranded for a year living on seal and polar bear. And during his first transit of the Northwest Passage, Roald Amundsen spent two years living among the Inuit on King William Land (now called Nunavut). Thus the Scandinavians were well acquainted with the diets of Polar cultures. But these were both situations dictated by the need for survival. No one would eat an Inuit diet by choice, right?

Well, here are a few names to chew on: John Rae, Frederick Schwatka, and Vilhjalmur Stefansson. All of them traveled thousands of miles through the Arctic between 1840 and 1920 employing the clothing, tools, and diet of the Inuit. Consuming a diet that was mostly fat and moderate in protein, clearly the lack of dietary carbohydrate didn't seem to hold them back. And in a particularly telling passage from his diary, Schwatka noted that it took him between two and three weeks to adapt to the Inuit diet, "after which prolonged sledge journeys are possible".

These observations suggest that the 'Achilles heel' of the carbohydrate-loading studies is their short duration (as in not enough time allowed for adaptation), and perhaps compounded by allowing their fear of fat to drive them to try to eat too much protein. To test this concept, we did a pair of studies a few decades ago[23, 76].

The first study involved six subjects given a very low energy (about 700 Calories per day) meat diet for 6 weeks, during which the average subject lost 25 pounds, which means that most of their daily energy came from body fat stores. Everybody was given supplements of sodium (3 grams per day), potassium, and a multivitamin. Before the diet, after one week, and after 6 weeks, each subject walked uphill on a treadmill until exhaustion. The average times on the treadmill were: 168 min, 130 min, and 269 min. Clearly one week did not allow enough time for the subjects to adapt to the low carbohydrate diet, and their exercise times decreased. After 6 weeks, however, there was a major rebound in performance. But before getting too excited by this huge increase, we need to point out that despite having each subject carry a backpack that brought them back to their starting weight, both their pulse rate and measured oxygen consumption indicated that they were doing less work at the same angle and speed on the treadmill during that final test. But that problem notwithstanding, these subjects obviously were not incapacitated by their 6 weeks on a very low carbohydrate intake.

To overcome this issue of improved efficiency with weight loss, and to get a more precise measure of the effects of dietary carbohydrate alone, we did a second study. This time we recruited 5 bicycle racers – lean and highly trained young men. Because they had little if any extra body fat to lose, we fed them a moderate protein (15% of energy) and very high fat diet (>80% of energy) patterned after what Stefansson ate in Bellevue Hospital in 1928. However because we were not interested in issues related to vitamins and minerals, we also gave them 5 grams per day of sodium, 1 gram of potassium, calcium and magnesium supplements, and a vitamin pill. And none of the meat was boiled!

At baseline, the average subject had a peak aerobic power of 5.1 liters of oxygen per minute and rode the stationary bike at 60% of this value for 147 minutes. This translates into a very impressive 900 Calories per hour for two and a half hours (with only water allowed during the ride). After four weeks on the Inuit diet, their peak aerobic power was unchanged at 5.0 liters per minute, and their duration at the same power output was 151 minutes (again no significant change from the high carb baseline values). What did change dramatically was muscle glycogen. Compared to baseline, they started the second ride with only half as much of it in their thigh muscles, and they only used a quarter as much to do the same amount of work. We also measured their bodies' use of blood sugar and total carbohydrate oxidation, and both of these were also dramatically reduced.

What did this prove? Well, if you're a cynic, you could say that 100 years later we just proved Frederick Schwatka right. But we also proved that, given the right amount of protein and minerals plus enough time (in this case, 4 weeks) for the human body to adapt, there is not a direct correlation between muscle glycogen content and work performance. However, this correlation between muscle glycogen content and performance is the key principal of the carbohydrate-loading construct, and our study demonstrated that it is only valid in the context of short term changes in diet. Thus, although the oft bandied truism that low carbohydrate diets necessarily impair physical performance remains alive in the minds of those who want to believe it, in reality it no longer has a basis in scientific fact.

Summary

Philosophers have been debating the meaning of scientific truth for thousands of years, and this chapter hasn't moved that boulder very far up the hill. Also, nothing we have presented here represents fraud. What we have presented are the contrasting fates of research data pertaining to low carbohydrate diets, and how this plays out in the context of a mainstream nutrition consensus that remains strongly biased against carbohydrate restriction.

All of the studies mentioned above were published more than 25 years ago, and in readily accessible and respected journals. So what we are not dealing with is the Warren & Marshall syndrome* – that 10 year window of hoping uncomfortable data will go away has long since expired. However we hope that we have provided you with some critical insight into how data is pitched by the medical media, and how the thoughtful reader can often find the truth between the lines.

We also hope that the issues we have discussed here bring a bit more clarity to future research. For example, defining a low carbohydrate diet as one under 100 grams per day of carbohydrate or less than 15% of daily energy intake would help, as would differentiating between ketogenic and non-ketogenic diets. Similarly, recognition that diets between 40-60% of energy as fat are fundamentally (and metabolically) different from those providing 70-80% as fat, and thus lumping them together under the single heading "high-fat" is misleading. And finally, the ongoing spate of short-term studies purporting to represent the long-term effects of carbohydrate restriction does a disservice to the science of this field (e.g., a recent 5-day study by Holloway et al.[97]). Avoiding these pitfalls would go a long way in resolving much of the confusion about low carbohydrate diets, and this clarity would serve the interests of those patients who stand to benefit from their use.

see sidebar in Chapter 14, Metabolic Syndrome chapter, page 177

Section 4

CLINICAL APPLICATIONS

Chapter 13

CLINICAL USE OF CARBOHYDRATE RESTRICTION: VERY LOW CALORIE AND LOW CARBOHYDRATE DIETS

Introduction

The evolution of carbohydrate restriction as a clinical tool over the last century has been essentially a search for sustainability. In the first half of the 1900s, the beneficial effects of total (or sub-total) starvation on conditions ranging from diabetes to epilepsy were observed. However, the negative effects of starvation on lean body mass and function necessarily curtails its use beyond brief periods. The exception to this pattern was the very high fat ketogenic diet developed by Wilder and Peterman for pediatric seizures, but this was considered by most practitioners to be too severe, and thus (perhaps inappropriately) superseded by drugs.

The 1970s brought us very low calorie diets (VLCD; aka protein sparing modified fasting) comprised of either common foods or prepared nutrient formulations. Most were used under medical supervision, including monitoring and provision of supplements. An exception to this practice of clinical monitoring and appropriate supplements led to the "Liquid Protein Diet" scandal – a problem of inadequate formulation and inadequate medical monitoring[98]. Typically providing between 300 and 800 Calories per day, VLCDs allowed severely obese patients to achieve rapid and major weight loss. But once the weight loss was achieved, the state

161

of nutritional ketosis induced by the carbohydrate restriction was relinquished (because most people then returned to a "balanced" maintenance diet), along with many of its associated metabolic benefits.

Parallel in time to the popularity of VLCDs, Dr. Robert Atkins promoted a less energy-restricted approach to a ketogenic diet. His focus was on keeping carbohydrate intake low enough to induce ketosis, but not to severely limit (or even count) calories. To achieve this, he advised individuals to eat protein and fat to satiety while keeping dietary carbohydrates low enough to maintain positive urine ketones. It was his view that this diet, including vegetables, limited fruit, and vitamin supplements, could be followed by the individual outpatient without close medical supervision unless there was a pre-existing complicating condition like diabetes or hypertension. For most patients, however, the Atkins diet tended to be only a temporary sojourn into nutritional ketosis, whether for want of sweets or want of approbation from their friends and doctor.

However, in these parallel few decades of the VLCD and Atkins diet, hundreds of studies were done, and we learned a great deal about carbohydrate restriction. Among these lessons are many which can contribute to the safe and sustainable use of carbohydrate restricted diets going forward.

Counting Calories vs Carbs

It was Dr. Atkins' contention that when most carbohydrate was removed from the diet, heavy people lose weight more effectively than by classic balanced calorie restriction. The mechanism was (and remains) hotly debated. Claims of reduced metabolic efficiency during nutritional ketosis remain unproven. Among other points against this is the fact that Steve Phinney's bike racers produced the same power output in testing on a stationary bike using the same oxygen consumption after adapting to the Inuit diet compared to their test on a high carb diet[23], leaving little room for metabolic inefficiency in this group of subjects.

But this argument over the mechanism of weight loss is an academic straw-man. In study after study, over the first 3-6 months, people randomized to a low carb diet eaten to satiety lose more weight and more body fat than those assigned to a low fat, calorie restricted diet. A credible mechanism to explain this is not hard to find – carbohydrates in our diet may offer a short-term sense of increased energy, but they offer little in the way of functional satiety.

The best example of this effect was reported by Dr. Guenther Boden[45] in an inpatient study of obese type-2 diabetics. After a week of eating a balanced diet to satiety, the subjects were given a low carbohydrate diet consisting of most of the same foods, with the exception that they were asked to limit their total daily carbohydrate intake to 20 grams. Over the next two weeks, their spontaneous nutrient intakes were carefully measured. Interestingly, the subject's average daily energy intake dropped from 3100 to 2100 Calories, and this was all due to the 'missing' carbs. Despite having the choice to eat more, the protein and fat intakes of these subjects remained relatively constant. And despite this 1000 Calorie per day deficit, their reported hunger, satisfaction, and energy levels did not change appreciably. What did change was their diabetes control – dramatically for the better. For more on this topic, see Chapter 15.

But this study was just 2 weeks long. What happens in the longer term? Well, the process of full metabolic adaptation to a low carbohydrate diet takes up to 6 weeks, so for the first few months, we would expect well-being and function to get better. But after many months and a major degree of weight loss, it is a normal response of the human body to try to limit its losses. This is typically achieved by eating more, but what? If dietary carbohydrate intolerance led to the choice of a low carbohydrate diet at the outset, why lift that restriction? In particular, why add back calories that promote fat storage but do not provide functional satiety? Accepting that protein is good for us only in moderation, the answer is *fat* (see Chapters 2 and 16). How much fat should you add as you approach weight maintenance? The simple answer: "let satiety rule".

Ketones – To Measure or Not

As noted in Chapter 1, nutritional ketosis is defined by serum ketones ranging from 0.5 up to 5 mM, depending on the amounts of dietary carbohydrate and protein consumed. In most people, the combined intake of 100 grams of carbohydrate and 100 grams of protein will drive serum ketones well below 0.5 mM. While there is nothing magical about having circulating ketones above this threshold level, it does have the practical value of providing the brain with a virtually limitless, fat-derived fuel source. This alternative fuel is eminently more sustainable, particularly in the insulin resistant or carbohydrate intolerant individual.

Within a few days of starting on carbohydrate restriction, most people begin excreting ketones in their urine. This occurs before serum ketones have risen to their stable adapted level because un-adapted renal tubules actively secrete beta-hydroxybutyrate and acetoacetate into the urine. This is the same pathway that clears other organic acids like uric acid, vitamin C, and penicillin from the serum.

Meanwhile, the body is undergoing a complex set of adaptations in ketone metabolism[99]. Beta-hydroxybutyrate and acetoacetate are made in the liver in about equal proportions, and both are initially promptly oxidized by muscle. But over a matter of weeks, the muscles stop using these ketones for fuel. Instead, muscle cells take up acetoacetate, reduce it to beta-hydroxybutyrate, and return it back into the circulation. Thus after a few weeks, the predominant form in the circulation is beta-hydroxybutyrate, which also happens to be the ketone preferred by brain cells (as an aside, the strips that test for ketones in the urine detect the presence of acetoacetate, not beta-hydroxybutyrate). The result of this process of keto-adaptation is an elegantly choreographed shuttle of fuel from fat cells to liver to muscle to brain.

In the kidney, this process of keto-adaptation is also complex. Over time, urine ketone excretion drops off, perhaps to conserve a valuable energy substrate (although urine ketone excretion never amounts to very many wasted calories). This decline in urine ketones happens over the same time-course that renal uric acid clearance returns to normal (discussed below) and thus may represent an adaptation in kidney organic acid metabolism in response to sustained carbohydrate restriction.

These temporal changes in how the kidneys handle ketones make urine ketone testing a rather uncertain if not undependable way of monitoring dietary response/adherence. Testing serum for beta-hydroxybutyrate is much more accurate but requires drawing blood, and it is expensive because it is not a routine test that doctors normally order.

A non-invasive alternative is to measure breath acetone concentration. Acetone is produced by the spontaneous (i.e., non-enzymatic) breakdown of acetoacetate. Because it is volatile, acetone comes out in expired air, and its content is linearly correlated with blood ketone levels. A number of businesses have developed prototype handheld devices to measure breath acetone, but at the time of this writing, nothing practical is on the market.

But whatever test is used, the key question is why do it? Many people are able to initiate and follow a low carbohydrate diet just fine without ever measuring ketones. Others, however, find an objective measure of nutritional ketosis to be reassuring. In some clinical settings, ketone testing is used as a measure of 'diet compliance'. While this may be useful in the short term to keep patients on track in a strictly regimented dietary program, it begs the question of how that individual's diet will be managed long term. For this purpose, the handheld breath acetone monitors under development hold some promise as a guidance tool put into the hands of the individual striving to find the right level of carbohydrate intake for long-term maintenance.

Biochemical changes (uric acid, acid/base, electrolytes, cholesterol mobilization)

There are often dramatic but wholly predictable changes that occur in blood chemistry values upon initiation of a low carbohydrate diet. As a result, and also due to the very limited food intakes of people following very low calorie diets, most clinics using them do routine blood tests over the first few months of dieting. Because of the greater intake of vegetables and total energy, a less restricted low carbohydrate diet such as Atkins raises fewer concerns in an otherwise healthy patient. Thus the choice of laboratory monitoring in this instance is left to one's physician, who should always be consulted by the patient before starting any weight loss regimen.

Early on in the VLCD era, hypokalemia (low blood potassium) was not uncommon, but once we learned to supply a modicum of sodium to avoid aldosterone-induced potassium wasting, this became a rare finding (limited usually to individuals with the concurrent use of diuretics). However, persistent hypokalemia unresponsive to sodium and potassium replacement can be a sign of underlying magnesium depletion[100]. Since serum magnesium is poorly correlated with intracellular magnesium, the best 'test' for magnesium depletion is a 20-day course of oral replacement (see Chapter 18) as long as the patient has normal renal function.

A very predictable change in serum chemistry is a sharp rise in uric acid concentration in the first week or two of carbohydrate restriction. As noted above, this is due to competition between circulating ketones and uric acid for renal tubular excretion. Put another way, uric acid rises in the blood not because the body is making more of it but because the kidneys temporarily clear less of it. Thus the blood level needs to rise in order for the same amount of it to be cleared by the kidney (because ketones are 'getting in the way'). Subsequent to this abrupt early rise in uric acid, within 4-6 weeks the level then falls back to or below its pre-diet level even if the dietary carbohydrate restriction and ketonemia continue. This is part of the body's ongoing adaptation to nutritional ketosis.

In the vast majority of patients, this rise in serum uric acid is completely benign and requires no intervention. In the minority of individuals predisposed to gout, however, wide swings in uric acid can trigger an attack. And this goes both ways – either the abrupt rise with diet initiation or the analogous abrupt fall if the ketonemia is reversed by breaking the carbohydrate restriction in the first few weeks, can act as a trigger. Most people with the genetic predisposition to gout know it long before they consider a low carbohydrate diet, so either preventative medication or prompt intervention at the first symptoms can usually pre-empt an attack. Also, because it is the rapid change in uric acid that is the primary trigger, once on a carbohydrate restricted diet, the patient with a history of gout should be counseled to avoid frequent cycling in and out of carbohydrate restriction (i.e., avoid 'going on and off the diet').

There is a persistent myth that nutritional ketosis results in clinically significant acidosis, despite overwhelming evidence to the contrary. Yes, the modest rise in serum ketones will shift serum chemistries a bit towards the acid end, but blood pH and serum bicarbonate values almost always remain well within the normal range. And the degree of this shift in pH is considerably less than that seen with just 5-7 days of total fasting, which is part of normal human physiology. Put another way, the buffering capacity of otherwise healthy humans is able to compensate across the full range of nutritional ketosis without any significant metabolic disturbance. Thus acid/base status does not need to be monitored during carbohydrate restriction in otherwise healthy individuals. In type-2 diabetics, however, if there is any question of an individual's insulin reserve (e.g., low serum insulin in the context of elevated blood glucose), monitoring of serum ketonemia and bicarbonate levels should be carefully considered.

There is one anomaly in clinical testing that physicians and patients should be aware of: a transient rise in serum total and LDL cholesterol that can occur with major weight loss. We reported this in 1991[101], and our research revealed the cause. It turns out that along with the triglyceride stored in adipose tissue, our fat cells also contains a small amount of dissolved cholesterol. After about 30 pounds of weight loss, the shrinkage of these cellular fat droplets proceeds to the point that some of this cholesterol has to be released into the serum. The amount of cholesterol involved is 100-200 mg per day in someone losing 2 pounds of adipose tissue per week. Interestingly, although this represents 'reverse transport' back to the liver, this cholesterol rise appears in the LDL fraction. But once a person's weight loss ceases, this expulsion of cholesterol stored in adipose tissue stops and serum LDL cholesterol returns to its new post-weight-loss baseline.

So if you or your patient experience a rise in serum LDL cholesterol as the scale passes 30 or more pounds of weight loss, don't panic. This is a sign that your body is dumping previously accumulated cholesterol. Since this situation typically lasts only a month or two, whereas it takes decades of elevated LDL cholesterol to cause blood vessel damage, the probability of any clinical risk is very small. Wait until your weight has stabilized in maintenance for a month or two and then test your LDL level again to be sure it has come back down.

Dietary Fat and Gallbladder Health

Although this transient rise in LDL cholesterol during major weight loss may look worrisome at first, it is a transient anomaly associated with the body's dumping cholesterol that had slowly accumulated in excess adipose tissue. The path of this cholesterol out of the body is as follows: it is taken up by the liver, secreted into bile which is stored in the gallbladder and then excreted via the gastrointestinal tract.

On its face, the 100-200 mg/day rate of clearance does not sound like much. After all, we typically eat more than 300 mg of dietary cholesterol per day. But most of the cholesterol we eat never gets absorbed, so an added 100-200 mg/day transiting the gall bladder is actually a fair amount. If someone who has already lost 30 pounds (thus triggering this efflux of cholesterol) proceeds to lose another 30 pounds over 3 months, that adds up to 10-20 grams of stored cholesterol the body has to get rid of.

Is this a problem? Well, not as long as the gallbladder gets regular signals to contract, coming in the form of cholecystokinin released by the upper small bowel in response to dietary fat. However, if dietary fat intake is low (under 30 grams per day) during rapid weight loss, the gallbladder doesn't get the signal to empty itself, and this cholesterol can build up and increase the risk of gallstone formation. Back in the VLCD era, some of the commercial formula diets were very low in fat, and their use was associated with a surprisingly high rate of gallstone formation[102]. However, if a meat/fish/poultry VLCD containing the associated natural fats was used, or 30 or more grams of fat was added to a liquid formula, new gallstone formation was rarely a problem.

Add one more item to the list of benefits of dietary fat. It protects your gallbladder from gallstones during major weight loss.

Level of Medical Monitoring

All individuals considering a low carbohydrate diet should consult their physician before starting. But unless there are significant abnormalities in cardiac, liver, kidney, or endocrine functions, frequent clinical monitoring may not be necessary as the diet proceeds. Clearly, medications for high blood pressure, fluid retention, glucose control, and dyslipidemia will need to be adjusted (usually this means withdrawn or decreased) as the diet proceeds – often sooner rather than later.

You Too, Doctor!

We know of more than one physician who has heard us give a talk and then launched themselves into a carbohydrate restricted diet. Typically we find out about it in the following type of conversation.

Them: "I love the weight loss on your diet, and I've been able to take myself off my (*blood pressure and/or diabetes*) medications, but how come I feel so lousy?"

Us: "Have you read our book? Are you drinking broth regularly?"

Them: "Book? Broth?"

Having read this far, you know why these are important for your health and well-being. And when you've finished the last chapter, you will be better equipped than most of your colleagues to manage people with this powerful clinical tool. But particularly if you are on medication for a weight-related condition, you need a physician (other than your mirror) monitoring your progress. If your personal physician isn't experienced in the use of low carbohydrate diets, Jimmy Moore (Chapter 21) has a service to help you find one who is, or you can just give your physician a copy of this book.

Role of Clinical Support

Independent of medical monitoring of one's low carbohydrate diet, there is an additional role for ongoing clinical support. Multiple studies with diets across a wide range of macronutrient compositions have shown that on average the amount of weight loss is positively correlated with the number of visits to a support group or clinic. This observation helps us understand the wide variations in the amounts of weight loss in studies using the same diets. But there is one important caveat – the support provided needs to be appropriate in content to the diet in question. If patients on a low carbohydrate diet attend a nutrition education group in which they are taught that high fat diets and saturated fats are bad, the net effect on that person's weight loss and well-being is likely to be negative.

List of Indications for Low Carbohydrate Dieting

In addition to its superior performance in achieving weight loss, there are a host of conditions that respond better to carbohydrate restriction than to other diet or lifestyle measures. Although many of these conditions are associated with insulin resistance, some others such as sleep apnea and seizures are not.

> insulin resistance/metabolic syndrome
> type-2 diabetes
> hypertension
> polycystic ovary syndrome (PCOS)
> gastroesophageal reflux disease (GERD)
> sleep apnea
> medication-resistant seizures

Summary

Weight loss induced by a well-formulated very low calorie diet can be dramatic, but VLCDs require closer medical supervision than a carbohydrate restricted diet providing more energy and a broader range of foods such as the Atkins Diet. Furthermore, the question of how to transition from a VLCD into a sustainable weight maintenance diet remains an issue, whereas it is a more natural transition from the early phases of Atkins to a low-carbohydrate maintenance energy intake. This is achieved by the simple expedient of maintaining the appropriate degree of carbohydrate restriction and adding more fat.

The beneficial effects associated with nutritional ketosis make this class of diets advantageous in the treatment of a number of clinical conditions. However, the often dramatic improvements in blood glucose control, blood pressure, and fluid retention require prompt adjustments in some medications. Therefore, as the complexity of these associated conditions is increased, closer medical attention and monitoring may be required.

Chapter 14

METABOLIC SYNDROME

Introduction

A chapter on metabolic syndrome might best be told as a "whodunit" detective story. The victims: approximately 64 million or 34% of adults with metabolic syndrome in the United States[103]. The perpetrator(s) of the crime: a cast of alleged suspects have been identified. Like any good mystery, a web of deception has been artfully cast to cloak the real culprit. For a while at least, the wrong suspect has been put in jail. If you're clever though, maybe you've already deduced the truly guilty party. But if not, in this chapter we'll lay out the key clues to the puzzle. And once deprived of his cloak, the villain, a well known player at the metabolic table, will be inescapably revealed.

Connecting the Dots –Solving the Crime

met·a·bol·ic (*adjective*) \\me-t-bä-lik\ - of, relating to, or based on metabolism.

syn·drome (*noun*) \sin-drōm\ - a group of signs and symptoms that occur together and characterize a particular abnormality or condition.

As the definitions imply, metabolic syndrome describes a collection of metabolic abnormalities. These derangements in combination are a harbinger of type 2 diabetes and cardiovascular disease. With any collection of symptoms, a good scientific detective asks whether there is a common cause. In the case of metabolic syndrome the common thread linking an ever growing constellation of abnormalities is insulin resistance. Insulin resistance is defined as a diminished response to a given concentration of insulin. While insulin resistance may be doing the dirty work at the cellular level, the ringleader of the metabolic syndrome crime syndicate is dietary carbohydrate. Since the inability to properly metabolize dietary carbohydrate is the direct result when insulin action is impaired, from a functional perspective, insulin resistance can be more accurately described as *carbohydrate intolerance*. When viewed in this context, carbohydrate restriction is a fully rational approach to treating the diverse factors that congregate in metabolic syndrome. Restricting carbohydrate is akin to arresting the crime boss – once you put the correct perpetrator in jail, everything else falls into place.

Syndrome X, Insulin Resistance Syndrome, and Metabolic Syndrome

Dr. Gerald Reaven is generally credited with making the observation that individuals with insulin resistance (as evidenced by hyperinsulinemia) showed common metabolic disturbances that significantly increased their risk of cardiovascular disease. In 1988 he termed this locus of symptoms 'syndrome X'[4]. Later he used the term 'insulin resistance syndrome', which more accurately reflected the underlying metabolic problem. The related term 'metabolic syndrome' was introduced by the Adult Treatment Panel III (ATP III) of the National Cholesterol Education Program. Reaven viewed the metabolic syndrome as a diagnostic tool to identify people at increased cardiovascular disease (CVD) risk based on the presence of specific criteria (see side bar). Regardless of the term used, the presence of insulin resistance is accepted as the underlying physiologic construct. Interestingly, Reaven recognized that the favored diet of the time – a low fat/high carbohydrate diet – would exacerbate the syndrome. This was self-evident from the title of his 1997 review paper[104] entitled *"Do high carbohydrate diets prevent the development or attenuate the manifestations (or both) of syndrome X? A viewpoint strongly against"*. Reaven was cognizant that "...low fat/high carbohydrate diets should be avoided in the treatment of syndrome X.", but few took heed of such warnings amidst the tsunami-like forces advocating in favor of fat restriction.

Metabolic Syndrome Defined[105]

You have metabolic syndrome if at least three of the following are present:

- Waist circumference: ≥40 inches (men) or ≥35 inches (women)

- Fasting triglycerides: ≥150 mg/dL

- HDL-C: <40 mg/dL (men) or <50 mg/dL (women)

- Blood pressure: ≥130/85 mm Hg or use of hypertensive medication

- Fasting glucose: ≥100 mg/dL or use of hyperglycemia medication

Competing Paradigms

Now that two decades have passed, why has carbohydrate restriction been ignored as an optional (if not preferred) treatment for metabolic syndrome? There are probably many reasons, but the 3-decade obsession with the diet-heart hypothesis, which focuses on reducing elevated LDL cholesterol (LDL-C), stands out. Note in the above table that LDL-C is not a factor in the diagnosis of metabolic syndrome. Thus dietary changes targeted at lowering LDL-C are different from those aimed at decreasing insulin resistance. From a treatment perspective, the diet-heart paradigm and metabolic syndrome represent separate abnormalities that increase CVD risk.

But at its heart, our medical research establishment is reductionist. It is clear that the authors of official dietary guidelines prefer to promote a simple unified message rather than explaining to the public that there is a logical choice of treatment options depending on the underlying cause of increased CVD risk. Thus the fact that dietary fat restriction is not the preferred diet therapy for metabolic syndrome hasn't sat very well with the mainstream medical consensus. As such, alternative approaches like low carbohydrate diets are ignored or condemned, despite the fact that their efficacy and safety are based on solid biochemical and metabolic grounds, supported by both scientific studies and clinical experience.

Carbohydrate Restriction – The Elephant in the Room

Over the last 20 years there have been tens-of-thousands of studies, review papers, and international scientific conferences focused on metabolic syndrome. How often can the words *carbohydrate restriction* be found in the thousands of peer-reviewed papers on metabolic syndrome? How often are these words uttered by researchers/clinicians at seminars about innovative treatment options for metabolic syndrome? Truthfully? Hardly ever!

This situation is so bizarre you might think copy editors are trained to remove these words from manuscripts and speakers forced to sign contracts to avoid mentioning *low* and *carbohydrate* in the same sentence. How did this level of cognitive dissonance become so pervasive across the medical field? And what compels otherwise reasonable healthcare professionals to ignore a potent tool for treating metabolic syndrome; opting instead for ineffective treatments based on low fat diets plus unproven drug combinations?

The explanation of this disconnect between data and consensus thinking is more behavioral than based upon clinical science. Clearly the research supporting low carbohydrate diets induces anxiety in many health professionals, who respond with various rationalizations to support the status quo. However, we also need to recognize that changes in the medical consensus rarely occur as an "Aha Moment". More commonly, change in response to scientific discovery is a long drawn out process that plays out in slow motion over a decade or more (see sidebar below).

A Classic Example of Resistance to Change: Peptic Ulcers and Helicobacter pylori

A recent example symbolic of the resistance to changing medical dogma is the treatment for upper GI (stomach and duodenal) ulcers.

Between 1984 and 1989, two Australian scientists (Drs. Warren and Marshall) published 5 papers in top quality journals that proved beyond a doubt that a bacterial infection (rather than too much acid) caused most ulcers in the stomach and duodenum. After that, year after year, doctors still treated ulcer patients with the same old ineffective diets and antacid drugs; and in severe cases, with major surgery. In 1988, frustrated by his inability to convince other scientists of his discovery, Dr. Marshall even infected himself with this bacterium and promptly developed a case of acute gastritis. Finally, about 1995, the medical consensus 'flipped', and the hot new treatment for ulcers became an antibiotic cocktail to eradicate *Helicobacter pylori*. Ten years after that, in 2005, Drs. Warren and Marshall were awarded the Nobel Prize.

Is this just a case of 'Monday morning quarterbacking'? Were the initial results of Warren and Marshall fuzzy or inadequately described? Were their results hard to confirm? If you've ever tried to tell your doctor about something new, perhaps you might not be surprised that the answers to all three questions are no, no, and no.

After their initial publications, it would have taken less than a year for another research group to reproduce their results and publish them. After all, the typical antibiotic cure only lasts 2 weeks, and healing begins within a few days. So at the very latest, confirmation of their hypothesis should have been published by 1990 and the treatment paradigm changed. Instead, the idea that bacteria could grow and cause problems in the acid environment of the stomach was discounted out-of-hand, if not ridiculed, by the experts. Why? Perhaps people regarded as experts become used to doing something one way for decades and don't like to admit that another way might be better. And because this is not an isolated phenomenon, for want of a better term, let's call this systemic reticence to accepting obvious change 'the Warren & Marshall Syndrome'.

Insulin Resistance Syndrome

In simple terms insulin resistance is a state in which a given concentration of insulin produces a less than expected biological effect. However, a key characteristic of metabolic syndrome is that the clinical expression of insulin resistance is variable, manifesting itself in different ways. This is a reflection of the multiple roles played by insulin throughout the body. Depending on where (e.g., skeletal muscle, liver, fat cells, etc.) and how much insulin resistance is present, the metabolic signs can vary widely between individuals and even within a given individual as the ability of various cells to respond properly to insulin deteriorates or improves. Moreover within any given cell there may be path-specific defects. That is, some insulin signaling pathways may be partially or fully resistant while others remain unaffected. Insulin resistance can therefore be a highly dynamic state producing a spectrum of phenotypes. This helps explain why metabolic syndrome is diagnosed by 3 or more out of 5 parameters, rather than by a single test yielding a single number. A brief review of insulin action and insulin resistance in various tissues is helpful to understand this range of markers that can present in metabolic syndrome.

What Causes Elevated Blood Glucose: Insulin Resistance in Skeletal Muscle or Liver?

Why did your bath overflow – was it because you forgot to turn off the faucet, or was the drain clogged?

Clogged Drain Theory: Insulin binding to its receptor on skeletal muscle induces a signaling cascade that results in translocation of intracellular glucose transporters (GLUT 4) to the sarcolemma (muscle cell membrane) and increased glucose uptake. Insulin resistance in muscle therefore results in decreased glucose uptake. A key defect appears to be an impaired ability of insulin to signal glucose transporters in muscle resulting in significantly decreased rates of glucose uptake and glycogen synthesis. The derangements in insulin-stimulated glucose uptake may result from accumulation of intramuscular fat which has been shown to inhibit activation of upstream elements in the insulin signaling cascade[106]. In this scenario, the insulin resistant muscle fails to increase glucose uptake resulting in accumulation of glucose in the blood stream.

Open Faucet Theory: An equally convincing case can be made for defects in hepatic insulin action as the driving force underlying high blood glucose[107]. The open faucet theory posits that the inability to suppress hepatic glucose output is the conductor of a poorly regulated glucose metabolism orchestra. In the fasting state, the liver is primarily responsible for secreting glucose to maintain a normal level the circulation. In the liver, insulin acts to inhibit glycogen breakdown and new glucose production, thus suppressing glucose output. In the insulin resistant liver there is an inability to suppress hepatic glucose output resulting in increased release of glucose into the circulation, even when it's not needed. As a compensatory mechanism, glucose uptake by the primary cells responsible for clearing glucose in the fasted state (e.g., brain, lean tissues, adipocytes, red blood cells) may be normal or even increased.

Either way, whether you have a clogged drain (impaired glucose uptake) or a wide open spigot (increased hepatic glucose output), the overflow of glucose (water) makes for a metabolic mess. In the fasted state the primary source of glucose entering the blood comes from the liver. The other major source of blood glucose is dietary carbohydrate. However, absorption of glucose from the intestines into the blood can be easily controlled by adjusting one's intake of carbohydrate. If the insulin resistant liver is already struggling to suppress its glucose output, providing an additional dietary source of glucose is completely irrational – think of aiming a fire hose into your already overflowing bathtub. Since progression to diabetes with life-threatening complications is one possible outcome, a more dangerous analogy than an overflowing bath might be in order. **Managing the metabolic mayhem in someone with insulin resistance by increasing dietary carbohydrate is like using a flame-thrower to fight a house fire.**

Insulin Resistance in Adipocytes

Adipocytes have a huge capacity for expansion (not only can each one can get bigger – we can also make more of them), and this excessive storage of adipose triglyceride is the basis for defining obesity. In no other time in history has the adipocyte's capacity for expansion been so challenged. The primary function of adipose tissue is to stockpile surplus fuel as triglycerides in lipid droplets and release that stored energy in the form of free fatty acids. However, within the last 15 years there has been an explosion of scientific papers revealing that adipocytes do much more than simply store and release fat. In addition, they produce a wide array of hormone-like substances called adipokines. These hormones are secreted into the circulation, exerting important effects on a host of physiologic processes (e.g., carbohydrate and fat metabolism, food intake, vascular and immune function, etc.). A key event was the discovery in 1994 that fat cells make the hormone leptin. This ushered in a new era in which the adipocyte is now viewed as a full-fledged endocrine cell. In addition to leptin, a host of additional adipokines produced in fat cells have been discovered and shown to play important roles in the development of insulin resistance.

It is helpful to take a step back and ask what goes wrong in obesity and metabolic syndrome from the perspective of the adipocyte. Expansion of adipose tissue does not happen spontaneously – it is in response to nutrient overload. Interestingly, despite nutrient excess and an expanding waistline, not all overweight people develop insulin resistance and metabolic syndrome. But two important things happen in those people who do. First, there appears to be a failure of adipose to fully accommodate the surplus fatty acids seeking a home, leading to ectopic fat accumulation in other organs such as muscle and liver. Second, there are qualitative and/ or quantitative changes in adipokine production, leading to changes in systemic insulin resistance. Let's briefly discuss each of these phenomena.

Fat accumulation in non-adipose tissues is largely due to insulin resistance in adipocytes. Insulin is the most important inhibitor of lipolysis, which is the hydrolysis of triglycerides to release fatty acids into the circulation. Its effects are immediate and exquisitely sensitive within the physiologic range of plasma insulin levels. The resultant changes in plasma fatty acid levels associated with low and high insulin levels can vary over a 10-fold range. Insulin resistance in the adipocyte results in an unregulated release of fatty acids that are subsequently taken up by other tissues and stored. An increase in muscle and liver fat is a well established feature of obese individuals with insulin resistance. Interestingly highly trained athletes with high levels of insulin sensitivity also pack more fat in their muscles (see side bar – Muscle Triglycerides and Insulin Resistance Paradox). And for the reader who likes technical detail, increased fatty acid derivatives in muscle and liver have been shown to increase kinases that phosphorylate IRS-1 on serine residues thereby inactivating this important upstream element in the insulin signaling cascade. This impaired insulin signaling leads to decreased GLUT 4 translocation and reduced muscle glucose uptake, setting up a vicious cycle that causes both greater fat production (lipogenesis) and insulin resistance.

Muscle Triglycerides and Insulin Resistance Paradox

A highly trained athlete and an obese (untrained) individual both have higher than normal plasma fatty acids and muscle triglycerides, yet the former has high insulin sensitivity while the latter is insulin resistant. Therein lies the paradox. If you delve into the exercise physiology literature you will quickly learn that one of the classic training adaptations is a shift to a greater proportion of fuel derived from fat during activity. The source of that fat may be derived from circulating fatty acids or muscle triglycerides. Thus, it makes sense that athletes would rev up their metabolic machinery to mobilize fatty acids from adipose tissue and increase local storage of triglyceride in muscle. In contradistinction the increase in plasma fatty acids in obesity is due to impaired insulin-induced inhibition of lipolysis (i.e., adipocyte insulin resistance). The increased release of fatty acids are taken up and deposited in muscle and other tissues. Do increased muscle triglycerides cause insulin resistance in the obese person but not in the athlete? Or is insulin resistance caused by something else and the fat buildup in untrained muscle just a symptom of the problem (aka, an epi-phenomenon)? These questions serve to emphasize an important point. Although insulin resistance has been a recognized problem for more than 50 years, its underlying cause is still not fully understood at the molecular level.

Thus this paradox. But there are some recent observations that give us hope of solving it. For one there is a significant difference in the flux through the muscle triglyceride pool. Athletes repeatedly break down triglycerides during exercise and rebuild them during recovery. To facilitate fat utilization, muscle triglycerides in trained individuals are localized near mitochondria within cells. In obesity, the muscle triglyceride pool is more inert and tends to be stored in droplets away from mitochondria. There is also a decreased number and size of mitochondria and overall reduced oxidative capacity in the untrained obese person. It is hypothesized that the mismatch between increased availability and decreased use of fat results in accumulation of lipid derivatives (e.g., diacylglycerol, ceramides) that garble the insulin signaling message causing insulin resistance. Paradox potentially explained.

Insulin resistance in adipocytes is also associated with a distorted secretion of adipokines. Several adipokines that promote hyperglycemia are increased (e.g., resistin, TNF-a, IL-6, RBP4) and those that promote insulin sensitivity decreased (e.g., adiponectin, visfatin, omentin). A low carbohydrate diet is more effective than a low fat diet at correcting the abnormal pattern of adipokine secretion in insulin resistance. For example, retinol binding protein-4 (RBP4) levels decreased in subjects on a low carbohydrate diet but not a low fat diet[56] (see side bar - RBP4: A Novel Adipokine Linked to Insulin Resistance).

Leptin levels in plasma are significantly increased in obesity and insulin resistance but the presence of leptin resistance prevents its normal actions (increased energy expenditure, decreased food intake, increased muscle and liver fatty acid oxidation). We recently showed a marked reduction in leptin in response to a low carbohydrate diet (-42%) compared to a low fat diet (18%)[56]. The greater decrease in leptin concentration persisted after normalization of values to account for the greater reductions in body mass and fat mass in the subjects consuming a low carbohydrate diet, suggesting an improvement in leptin sensitivity. Emerging evidence has shown proinflammatory effects of leptin implicating it in the pathogenesis of inflammatory conditions[108], and thus lower leptin is consistent with an overall anti-inflammatory effect of carbohydrate restriction (discussed later in this chapter).

RBP4: A Novel Adipokine Linked to Insulin Resistance

In 2005, an article in the journal Nature identified RBP4 as a potent adipokine[109]. Since then, a number of studies have confirmed and elucidated its role in metabolic syndrome. RBP4 is expressed primarily in liver and adipocytes. Genetic deletion of RBP4 enhances insulin sensitivity, and over-expression causes insulin resistance in mice. In humans, elevation of serum RBP4 is highly correlated with insulin resistance and metabolic syndrome components suggesting that RBP4 may be an important contributor to cardiovascular risk. Therefore, we hypothesized that RBP4 levels would be reduced by carbohydrate restriction. Overweight/obese non-diabetic subjects with metabolic syndrome were randomized to either a very low carbohydrate ketogenic diet or a low fat diet for 12 weeks[56]. Compared to subjects consuming low fat, subjects on the low carbohydrate diet showed improved glycemic control, insulin sensitivity and atherogenic dyslipidemia (decreased triglyceride, increased HDL-C, and increased LDL particle size). Serum RBP4 levels were reduced more in subjects on the low carbohydrate diet (-20%) compared to the low fat diet (+5%) (P=0.02). For all subjects, the change in amount of dietary carbohydrate intake correlated with the change in RBP4; the correlation was stronger in subjects on the low carbohydrate diet (r=0.54). The absolute and percent changes in RBP4 correlated with weight loss, fat loss, and improvement in glucose, insulin, triglycerides, and the quantity of small LDL particles.

These findings link the role of RBP4 in insulin resistance with studies showing a tight connection between carbohydrate restriction and features of metabolic syndrome. Dietary interventions that do not reduce carbohydrate intake may be ineffective in lowering serum RBP4, even when significant weight loss is achieved. In addition to improvement in markers of metabolic syndrome, elevated serum RBP4 may be an important pathogenic feature of metabolic syndrome whose reduction is tightly correlated with reduced dietary carbohydrate intake.

Insulin Resistance and Dyslipidemia

The primary abnormalities seen in blood lipids with metabolic syndrome are varying combinations of elevated plasma triglyceride, low HDL-C, and a predominance of small LDL particles. Insulin resistance in adipocytes and liver facilitate this disturbed lipid pattern. In addition to decreasing hepatic glucose output, insulin also inhibits hepatic triglyceride secretion by suppressing VLDL output. Thus insulin resistance in the liver results in overproduction and release of both glucose and triglyceride into the circulation. The process is exacerbated by greater delivery of plasma fatty acids to the liver as a result of adipocyte insulin resistance. Hepatic re-esterification of fatty acids and subsequent over-production of large triglyceride-rich VLDL ensue. This, combined with impaired clearance of plasma triglyceride, results in a constant state of hypertriglyceridemia in both the postabsorptive and postprandial periods. This in turn leads to the exchange of triglyceride in VLDL for cholesteryl ester in LDL. The resulting triglyceride-rich LDL particle is a preferred substrate for hepatic lipase and lipoprotein lipase and therefore becomes the source of small, dense LDL. Similarly, triglyceride-rich HDL is hydrolyzed by lipoprotein lipase resulting in the generation of smaller HDL particles that are rapidly removed from the circulation. In this way elevated triglyceride resulting from disruption in insulin function plays a central role in regulating the atherogenic dyslipidemia of metabolic syndrome.

Insulin Resistance and Low-Grade Inflammation

A large body of research has implicated elevated inflammation in metabolic syndrome and the pathogenesis of diabetes, heart disease, and other chronic diseases[110]. What is the link between insulin resistance and increased constituitive inflammation? There are several theories, but first it is informative to explore the effects of insulin on inflammatory pathways. Insulin normally exerts anti-inflammatory effects. For example, insulin decreases gene expression of several inflammatory transcription factors in leukocytes inducing a broad spectrum anti-inflammatory effect. In the presence of inflammation induced by endotoxin or diabetes, acute increases in insulin suppress the concentration of inflammatory mediators. Insulin sensitizing drugs have been shown to exert anti-inflammatory effects. Thus as long as cells are responsive to insulin, inflammation appears to remain in check. Impairment of insulin action, however, results in increased inflammation and explains why metabolic syndrome is associated with low-grade inflammation. Just as insulin resistance induces inflammation, several studies have implicated inflammatory mediators in promoting insulin resistance. Understanding the origins of the inflammation is imperative to prevent this potential vicious cycle from escalating. It also opens the door to understanding how best to manage elevated inflammation.

What is inflammation? Frankly, it might be easier to explain the meaning of life. Why? Because there is an intricate web of interacting hormones, cytokines, and oxy-lipids (eicosanoids) that constitute what we loosely call the body's immune system. One view is that chronic inflammation is the net effect of repeated exposures to substances that trigger an immune response. For example celiac disease is a chronic inflammatory condition of the small intestines characterized by an aberrant immune response to gluten. Removal of gluten from the diet results in rapid remission of the inflammation and intestinal symptoms.

In an insulin resistant state, such as metabolic syndrome, the substance constantly irritating and provoking the body is carbohydrate. Carbohydrate ingestion and acute hyperglycemia activate a host of inflammatory and free radical-generating pathways[111, 112]. Some of these include: stimulation of NAPDH oxidase, superoxide generation by leukocytes, TNF-a production, and activation of NF-kB which regulates the transcriptional activity of over 100 pro-inflammatory genes. Consistent with the notion that carbohydrate can aggravate inflammatory balance, many studies have reported that low carbohydrate diets decrease markers of constituitive inflammation[29, 113].

Insulin Resistance in Endothelial Cells

Endothelial cells line the entire circulatory system, providing a barrier between blood and the vessel wall. It has become increasingly apparent that endothelial cells produce several vasoactive substances and other inflammatory mediators that regulate vasomotor function and vascular health. Endothelial cells have insulin receptors that trigger classic insulin signaling pathways very similar to skeletal muscle. Insulin resistance in endothelial cells has been shown to be due to impairment in the phosphatidyl inositol 3-kinase-dependent signaling pathway that leads to production of the potent vasodilator nitric oxide. To make matters worse, insulin also increases secretion of the vasoconstrictor endothelin-1 and this insulin signaling pathway appears to remain intact in the presence of insulin resistance[114]. This is an example of pathway specific insulin resistance that in this case inhibits a potent dilator and stimulates a strong constrictor. In other words, an insulin resistant endothelial cell is like driving a car with a broken accelerator and the parking brake on.

Carbohydrate Intake, Glucose and Insulin

Dietary carbohydrate is a direct source of blood glucose. Therefore restriction in dietary carbohydrate intuitively leads to fewer fluctuations in blood glucose. Ingesting carbohydrate, especially rapidly digested forms, stimulates a rapid increase in insulin from the pancreas. Continued stimulation by insulin, as with most hormones, has been shown to down-regulate the insulin response in a host of tissues (i.e., adipose tissue, liver, cardiac, smooth and skeletal muscles)[115, 116]. This insulin-stimulated insulin resistance is reversible by decreasing tissue exposure to insulin.

Insulin resistance itself leads to compensatory hyperinsulinemia, initiating a positive feedback loop (a vicious cycle). At some point the individual signs and symptoms of metabolic syndrome will emerge, especially under constant stress to increase insulin (i.e., carbohydrate intake). Depending on carbohydrate intake and the level of carbohydrate tolerance, the metabolic syndrome markers can and usually do change quickly, for the better or worse. One of the metabolic rationales for carbohydrate restriction is that reduced dietary glucose leads to better insulin control which disrupts the stimulus promoting insulin resistance (i.e., it breaks the vicious cycle). Studies using carbohydrate-restricted diets consistently show better glucose and insulin control and increased insulin sensitivity, both in healthy populations[56] and especially in patients with pre-existing metabolic syndrome or type-2 diabetes[45].

Defining Carbohydrate Intolerance

Given this emerging understanding of dietary carbohydrate as both an underlying cause and exacerbator of extant insulin resistance, it is instructive to view insulin resistance, metabolic syndrome and type-2 diabetes as carbohydrate intolerant conditions. What does carbohydrate intolerance mean? In medicine, intolerance is characterized by extreme sensitivity (in a negative way) or allergy to a drug, food, or other substance. Common forms of food intolerances include abnormal responses to lactose and gluten ingestion that in both cases promptly improve when the offending substances are restricted in the diet. In a person intolerant to carbohydrate, there is an exaggerated glucose and insulin response to a given amount of carbohydrate ingested.

A more insidious manifestation of insulin resistance, because of impaired glucose uptake into muscle, is a propensity to divert ingested carbohydrate to the liver where it is converted to fat. Metabolism of carbohydrate through de novo lipogenesis leads to increased plasma triglycerides and dyslipidemia. This is partially driven by a down-regulation of the insulin response and decreased glucose uptake in extrahepatic tissues.

Less well understood is how dietary carbohydrate impacts immune function and inflammatory mechanisms, but another facet of carbohydrate intolerance is likely an aberrant inflammatory response to carbohydrate intake. Clearly the normal response to carbohydrate in insulin sensitive tissues is disturbed in insulin resistance, which subscribes to the definition of intolerance. Put simply, consuming too much carbohydrate is like metabolic kryptonite if you already have insulin resistance.

Carbohydrate Restriction: the Rosetta Stone for Preventing and Treating Metabolic Syndrome

Reviewing the literature, one finds a remarkable consistency in studies that have compared low fat and low carbohydrate diets on markers of metabolic syndrome. Low carbohydrate diets perform at least as well, and usually better than low fat diets[56, 117, 118]. This includes improvements in triglycerides, HDL-C, LDL particle size, glucose, and insulin. In studies where the level of carbohydrate restriction is very low, there are often striking differences. For example, the benefits of carbohydrate restriction on markers of metabolic syndrome have been observed in normal or overweight individuals with or without the presence of metabolic syndrome, although the magnitude of improvement is often greatest in individuals with insulin resistance and frank type-2 diabetes.

The benefits of carbohydrate restriction are also apparent whether weight loss occurs or not, suggesting it is the reduction in dietary carbohydrate, not calories or body fat mass per se, that is responsible for the improved metabolic outcomes. That the signs of metabolic syndrome are precisely the ones targeted by diets that restrict carbohydrate should not be surprising, since the literature is rich in studies supporting this idea, yet there has been a palpable reluctance to make this explicit connection. We published a review paper in 2004[118] titled "Carbohydrate restriction improves the features of metabolic syndrome: metabolic syndrome may be defined by the response to carbohydrate restriction" in which we collected information in the literature supporting the notion that the major metabolic problems are specifically ameliorated by reduction in dietary carbohydrate, and thus had an advantage over low fat diets. However, this review seems to suffer from the Warren & Marshall Syndrome, as it has neither been refuted nor accepted by mainstream government or professional medical organizations.

Summary

Metabolic syndrome encompasses a widening circle of metabolic derangements that arise from a down-regulation of insulin-response in different cells. Given the established close connection between dietary carbohydrate and insulin physiology, carbohydrate restriction represents a powerful tool capable of inducing a unique metabolic state that targets the underlying cause of insulin resistance and metabolic syndrome. In view of the poor track record of low fat, high carbohydrate diets in controlling our current epidemic of obesity and diabetes, plus the limited impact of both pharmacologic and even exercise interventions on metabolic syndrome markers, a well-formulated low carbohydrate diet offers an effective alternative for the millions of Americans suffering from this reversible condition.

So what is the verdict in this 'whodunit' case? The culprit is our excessive intake of insulin-stimulatory dietary carbohydrates, especially simple sugars and refined starches. Lock enough of them up permanently, and the metabolic crime spree will end. Good work detective – metabolic syndrome solved – case closed!

Chapter 15

TREATING TYPE-2 DIABETES
AS CARBOHYDRATE INTOLERANCE

Introduction

The hallmark of type-2 diabetes is insulin resistance, but the actual biology of its underlying cause remains obscure. However, the two best predictors of who will develop diabetes in a cohort of healthy subjects are biomarkers of inflammation (such as c-reactive protein [CRP] and interleukin-6 [IL-6]) and the biomarker of lipogenesis, palmitoleic acid (POA) in the serum cholesteryl ester fraction. So absent a better explanation of the root cause of this disease, it makes sense that it is driven by inflammation and the diversion of dietary carbohydrate into secondary disposal pathways. Furthermore, as we discussed in Chapter 9, these two processes are mechanistically linked together by increased ROS production damaging membranes, leading to insulin resistance.

If this is indeed a primary underlying pathophysiology of type-2 diabetes, then it follows that the optimum treatment of type 2 diabetes is reduced dietary carbohydrate intake. After all, very low carbohydrate diets reduce the body's level of inflammation, particularly in conditions such as metabolic syndrome in which it is typically elevated. And restricting carbohydrate intake reduces the total burden of glucose needing disposal, taking the pressure off of secondary disposal pathways like lipogenesis.

On the continuum of insulin resistance, impaired glucose tolerance and more generally metabolic syndrome often progress to overt type-2 diabetes, and therefore the latter represents a more severe form of carbohydrate intolerance. This may mean that in its long-term management, daily carbohydrate intake has to be kept lower in a type-2 diabetic than in someone with less severe insulin resistance. But it also means that a well formulated low carbohydrate diet will tend to produce striking improvements when implemented in type-2 diabetics.

So what evidence is there that this approach actually works? That depends upon who you ask. The American Diabetes Association has been strongly against low carbohydrate diets for decades, but recently altered their position to acknowledge that there may be a role for diets lower in carbohydrate than they have previously been advocating[119].

And then there is clinical experience and the published literature. Let's start with a clinical case. This case was the first patient that Steve Phinney ever put on a ketogenic diet, occurring during his medical residency under the direction of Dr. Ethan Sims at the University of Vermont. The outcome for this patient was so remarkable that it helped shape Steve Phinney's research career.

Clinical Case: Type-2 Diabetic with Congestive Heart Failure

(Medical Center Hospital of Vermont, Mary Fletcher Unit, October 1975)

TR was an obese male in his late 40's with a long history of type-2 diabetes. He was admitted to hospital for management of his severely elevated blood sugar in anticipation of elective surgery to remove a large calcified gallstone. On exam, he had severe lower extremity edema resistant to high dose furosemide. His labs revealed normal kidney function but fasting glucoses between 250 and 300 mg/dl. For 3 days, we tried the standard treatment of an 1800 Calorie ADA diet, oral sulfonylurea agents, and 4 dose per day insulin; but TR's clinical response to these measures was unsatisfactory. Neither his severe edema nor his markedly elevated glucose values improved very much. The patient continued to have orthopnea (shortness of breath when lying flat), and his severe edema limited his activity to a bed-to-chair existence.

On the 4th day, Dr. Sims mentioned that one of his former research fellows, Dr. Bruce Bistrian, was studying a very low carbohydrate diet to manage type-2 diabetes at Harvard. So we cobbled together a research protocol and put TR on this diet, which consisted of modest portions of lean meat, fish, and poultry providing 90-100 g/d of protein in a total of 600 Calories, plus about 10 grams of carbohydrate. The diet was supplemented with potassium, trace minerals, and vitamins.

Within 48 hrs, TR's blood glucose values began to plummet towards normal, allowing us to cut way back on his insulin dosage. In addition, his urine output went up sharply, resulting in weight losses of 5 pounds per day. By the end of a week on the diet, his fasting blood glucoses were under 120, we had stopped all of his injected insulin, he'd lost 30 pounds and his edema had completely resolved despite our reducing his furosemide dose from 320 to 40 mg/day. But most striking of all, the patient was out of bed and pacing laps up and down the hospital ward, claiming that he'd not felt this good in years, and asking to be discharged so he could go fishing.

A few days later, the patient was discharged home on the same diet. He lost another lost 50 pounds in 5 months, and was then readmitted to have his cholecystectomy, which was performed without complications or recurrent signs of his diabetes.

Very Low Calorie Ketogenic Diets in Type-2 Diabetes

Concurrent with this and subsequent cases that we generated in Vermont, Dr. Bistrian completed a series of seven closely monitored cases in Cambridge/Boston[120]. It was his very low carbohydrate ketogenic (VLCKD) diet protocol that we used in the case study above. All seven of the subjects in his published report were obese, insulin-using type-2 diabetics, and all were able to be withdrawn from insulin therapy (up to 100 units per day) in an average of 7 days after starting the VLCKD. All of these subjects went on to lose a considerable amount of weight, an achievement that is decidedly uncommon in diabetics who are using injected insulin.

The pivotal issue with this use of the VLCKD in type-2 diabetics was their dietary management once the desired weight loss was achieved. While very effective in achieving weight loss, a diet providing 600-800 Calories per day was clearly unsustainable in the long run. For some of these formerly obese patients who were severely diabetic at the outset (like the case history above), their insulin resistance improved so much after major weight loss that they could transition to a low-glycemic index mixed diet without the return of overt diabetes. But for many others, the re-introduction of even a moderate amount of dietary carbohydrate promptly resulted in elevated serum glucose values despite maintaining a significant weight loss. And for all of these patients, there lurked the problem of eventual weight regain, and with it increasing insulin resistance.

Clearly the key to the long-term success in managing type 2 diabetes with carbohydrate restriction has been figuring out how to safely and effectively maintain the carbohydrate restriction into the weight maintenance phase of the diet. From the safety perspective, it helps a lot that we have demonstrated that blood levels of saturated fats decline despite eating a high fat, energy maintenance diet[30], and also that inflammation biomarkers (like IL-6 and CRP that are associated with the cause of type-2 diabetes) are also significantly reduced. These factors, along with the often dramatic improvements in serum triglycerides, HDL cholesterol, and LDL particle size, present a picture of across-the-board improvements in known health risk predictors when patients (diabetic or not) adhere to a well-formulated carbohydrate restricted diet.

But this then brings us to the question: what is the proper diet formulation for the formerly diabetic individual on carbohydrate restriction going into the maintenance phase? The answer, as we have emphasized throughout this book, is that it is a diet adequate in energy, moderate in protein, and high in fat. However, the key question is: how much does one need to restrict carbohydrate long-term? Or put another way, how does the individual know if s/he is eating too much carbohydrate?

One way to assess this would be to monitor blood glucose values as one's weight loss slows, where the goal is to hold carbohydrates down to that level that keeps blood glucose in the normal range. While this is, in and of itself, an excellent therapeutic success for someone who was formerly a type-2 diabetic, it may not be enough for that individual to stay normo-glycemic long term. Why might this be? Isn't keeping your blood sugar normal evidence that your diabetes is in complete remission?

The answer is that it's great to have normal blood sugars, but this will only last if you also keep off the lost weight. For this, success at maintaining your weight loss may take a greater degree of carbohydrate restriction that that needed to maintain blood sugar control. Why? Because, at the most basic level, successful weight maintenance requires not having blood sugar diverted into secondary disposal pathways like lipogenesis. To monitor this, you can monitor blood triglycerides and adjust dietary carbohydrate to keep them low. In addition, we are working on developing a test for POA levels as a more direct way to monitor the body's rate of lipogenesis (discussed in Chapters 9 and 11).

Hepatic Glucose Output With Varying Carbohydrate Restriction

Along with insulin resistance and accelerated lipogenesis, another hallmark of abnormal metabolism associated with type-2 diabetes is increased hepatic glucose output. Normally the liver releases glucose to prevent hypoglycemia, whereas glucose output by the liver goes way down when blood glucose values are elevated. But in type-2 diabetes, the insulin-resistant liver inappropriately keeps on dumping glucose into the circulation in spite of high blood sugar levels, making blood glucose control that much more difficult.

In 1996, Dr. Barry Gumbiner and colleagues published a seminal study showing the effects of carbohydrate restriction on hepatic glucose output in obese subjects with type-2 diabetes[121]. They constructed two VLCD's with the same protein and total energy (650 Calories), but one provided an average of 24 grams per day of carbohydrate, whereas the other contained 94 grams of carbs. The subjects followed each diet in random order for 3 weeks, and the average total weight loss was 11 kg over the 6-week study.

Interestingly, despite the big difference in carbohydrate intakes between the two diets, the rates of weight loss were the same for the two diets. However fasting blood sugars, while coming down dramatically on both diets, were consistently lower during the lower carbohydrate diet. The lower carb diet also raised serum ketones about twice as much as the higher carb diet. Both diets significantly reduced hepatic glucose output, but the more ketogenic diet reduced it by 22% more.

When the data from both diets were analyzed together, Dr. Gumbiner reported a strong and highly significant negative correlation between blood ketones and hepatic glucose output. What this means, quite simply, is that two diets identical in protein and total calories had distinctly different effects on type-2 diabetics, based solely upon their differing carbohydrate contents. Thus, despite similar rates of weight loss, the diet providing 24 grams/day of carbohydrate resulted in better diabetes control than the one providing 94 grams/day. And the negative correlation between serum ketones and hepatic glucose output indicates that the nutritional ketosis induced by the greater degree of carbohydrate restriction more effectively reversed underlying hepatic insulin resistance.

As an aside, it is interesting to track the fate of this paper and its novel findings since it was published in 1996. Although it has not been refuted, this paper has been cited in the medical literature just 12 times, even as the prevalence of type-2 diabetes is increasing in the developed and developing nations at a torrid pace. It is hard to know precisely why this paper has been relegated to the doghouse, but perhaps it is because ketones and nutritional ketosis continue to be casually discounted by both dietetic and medical educators, many of whom lack a basic understanding of the role ketones play in human energy metabolism. For a bit more in-depth look at some of the polarity that exists between research data and consensus experts, see Chapter 12.

A Sustainable and Effective Ketogenic Diet for Type-2 Diabetes

Not all clinically relevant studies need to be randomized or placebo-controlled trials. As with the 1976 Bistrian study[120] just described and Boden's recent study[45], a recently published pair of papers from Kuwait[122, 123] offers some important and clinically useful observations. These papers report the results from a large clinical practice managing adults with severe obesity. A cohort of 185 subjects was identified as potential candidates for the study, of whom 66 agreed to participate. The mean initial BMI of the subjects was 39 (i.e., as a group, they were severely obese). Baseline serum analysis was used to divide the cohort into two sub-groups: those with (n=35) and without (n-31) severe dyslipidemia. The 'dyslipidemic group', although not identified as diabetic, also had a mean baseline fasting glucose of 9.4 mM (169 mg/dl), and thus was composed predominantly of individuals with either severe metabolic syndrome or overt diabetes.

The same diet was used for both cohorts, consisting of meat, poultry, fish, eggs, and cheese plus vegetables providing 80-100 g/d of protein and 20 grams of total carbohydrate. To this was added 5 tablespoons (600 Calories) per day of olive oil used in cooking and on salads. Including the fats inherent in the protein sources, this diet provided 1200-1500 Calories per day. After 12 weeks, the carbohydrate restriction was increased to 40 grams per day, allowing inclusion of a wider list of vegetables, olives, avocados, and berry fruits. Beyond this, no further expansion of diet choices was recommended for one year.

Of the initial 66 subjects, 49 remained in the study after 56 weeks, including 26 of the initial 35 with dyslipidemia. The mean weight loss in this sub-group was 27 kg, with 11 kg of this weight loss occurring between months 6 and 12. At 8 weeks, mean fasting blood glucose had fallen from 9 to 6 mM (the upper limit of normal), from which point it declined further to 5 mM at 56 weeks. In addition, LDL cholesterol declined significantly, triglycerides were reduced 3-fold, and HDL cholesterol increased by 63%. Similar weight loss and improved (albeit not as dramatic) blood lipids were observed in the non-dyslipidemic group. When the last observation from the 17 dropouts was carried forward to the 56-week mark, these dramatic changes were not significantly attenuated, which means that the diet had a uniform beneficial effect on the subjects if they completed the study or not.

As this was not a randomized trial, there may have been some selection bias in enrolling subjects. But that notwithstanding, the remarkable total weight loss by this group, plus the fact that the weight loss continued through the second 6 months of the study, is striking. But the most profound change observed in this report was that 26 of the initial 35 'dyslipidemic' group normalized their markedly elevated blood glucose values within 2 months and remained at non-diabetic glucose levels for the rest of the year of observation. Simply put, here is an example of a cohort of type-2 diabetics who had their disease put into complete remission for a year (with an open-ended option to continue on this diet), during which time they lost and maintained a dramatic amount of weight while markedly improving severe dyslipidemia.

There is no other combination of diet and/or drugs that has been demonstrated to achieve this degree of weight loss plus diabetic control in a sizeable outpatient cohort. If the standard low fat, calorie restricted diet plus oral agents and insulin had been employed with the vigor necessary to achieve this level of glucose control in outpatients, the price of the glucose control would have been an increase in weight and further elevated triglycerides. Why? Because weight gain has been a consistent observation whenever diabetic groups are encouraged to pursue 'tight control', and this is easily understood due to insulin's potent role as a storage hormone. In addition, 'tight control' achieved by insulin plus insulin stimulating/ sensitizing medications carries an increased risk of hypoglycemic episodes, which are not benign. However, the opposite effect is achieved by removing most of the carbohydrate from the diets of individuals who are severely insulin resistant, facilitating better glucose homeostasis while at the same time allowing the body to access its excess fat reserves. Thus this study demonstrates excellent blood glucose control, major weight loss, plus dramatic improvement in blood triglycerides on a low carb regimen.

Critics of this paper point to the magnitude of the reported weight loss and ask how this study was able to achieve more than triple that reported in published randomized controlled trials, and how the subjects could sustain the diet for a year with continuing weight loss. There is no simple answer to this criticism, because clearly there were a number of potential contributing factors. One factor was the severe obesity of this cohort. Starting at a BMI of 39, they had a lot of weight to lose.

A second factor was precisely the fact that this was not a randomized trial. The clinic in which the study was done has used this diet, found it effective, and believes in its safety and efficacy. This message is not lost on patients and/or research subjects. If a study is done employing a diet that the research physician or dietitian is not comfortable with, this is effectively communicated to the subjects, and the resultant outcome is compromised. It is not uncommon to hear consensus experts say "We tried that diet, and it didn't work". But what do you expect when you ask a person to give up some of their favorite foods and change habits ingrained over decades, yet at the same time communicate to them (whether verbally or non-verbally) that you really don't believe these difficult life-style changes are necessary or safe?

A third factor, and one probably equally as important as the above two, is the prescription of added fat to the diet from its outset. This communicates to patients that dietary fat is good for them and a necessary part of their diet. While protein has an important role in satiety during weight loss dieting, it is nowhere near as effective as fat. So by adding 600 Calories of olive oil to their daily diet, individuals who were burning upwards of 3000 Calories per day achieved added satiety while still maintaining a sizeable energy deficit.

And finally, the addition of carbohydrate back into the diet in this cohort was strictly limited to a maximum of 40 grams. Biologically, particularly for individuals with severe insulin resistance or type-2 diabetes, this keeps them in ketosis and avoids their crossing back over that threshold (defined by Dr. Gumbiner's study[121]) where hepatic glucose output increases and diabetic control is lost. Also important from a behavioral perspective, telling a person that they can progressively add more and more dietary carbohydrate means that they don't need to make their peace with not having it. All they need do is wait a few months (or even just until dark, when no one is looking!) Why are we then surprised when the average research subject in an outpatient carbohydrate restriction study given unlimited, open-ended access to carbohydrate foods totaling more than 100 grams per day starts regaining weight after 6 months?

Does this mean that everyone on a carbohydrate restricted diet needs to stay under 40 grams per day? Of course not! Individuals vary tremendously in their degrees of carbohydrate tolerance. But in the context of this chapter about managing type-2 diabetes, we need to remember that insulin resistance is a hallmark of carbohydrate intolerance. For many patients starting out with type-2 diabetes, even after major weight loss and maintaining normal blood sugars for months, their underlying carbohydrate intolerance remains. That in turn means that these individuals will need to maintain a tight level of carbohydrate restriction (be it 30 grams, 60, or 90) for decades (not just a few months) to remain healthy and non-diabetic.

It's a bit simplistic but helpful to view a low carbohydrate diet as the 'natural' nutrient mix that a type-2 diabetic's body is wired to handle. By restricting the primary source of the problem, everything gets better. If you get a thorn in your foot...it hurts, so you remove the thorn as fast as possible. You don't take a pain killer and then keep walking on it hoping it will get better. A high carbohydrate diet is the proverbial 'metabolic thorn' for diabetics, and cutting down on dietary carbohydrate intake stops the metabolic pain at its source.

Summary

There are hundreds of published studies pertaining to the use of carbohydrate restricted diets in type-2 diabetes, some of them going back over a century. It has not been the goal of this chapter to perform a comprehensive review of this vast literature, but rather to focus on a few studies that reveal important aspects of developing a safe, effective, and sustainable clinical tool for the management of type-2 diabetes.

The three key take-away points made above can be summarized as follows:

1. Although carbohydrate-restricted diets can be dramatically effective in correcting blood glucose and lipid disorders associated with type-2 diabetes, in many if not most patients, these improvements do not last very long after the carbohydrate restriction ends. Thus there is little role for this type of diet to be employed in the management of diabetes in the short term. For most diabetic patients choosing to start a low carbohydrate diet (or being encouraged to start one by a health care professional), the individual needs to be aware of the likelihood that some degree of carbohydrate restriction will have to become a regular part of their ongoing healthy lifestyle.

2. The degree of carbohydrate restriction needed to achieve one's goals of weight loss and diabetes control will vary greatly among individuals. It may also vary within any one individual as well, in the sense that the degree of restriction to promote weight loss may be less strict or different from that needed to optimally control the metabolic abnormalities associated with type-2 diabetes. For example, Dr. Gumbiners' subjects on his higher carbohydrate diet lost the same amount of weight but had less effective suppression of their high blood glucoses and hepatic glucose output. Seen from this perspective, maintaining a state of moderate nutritional ketosis (1-2 mM serum beta-hydroxybutyrate) may be a beneficial biomarker of efficacy, and this usually requires holding daily carbohydrate intakes in the 20-50 g/day range.

3. The ability to sustain such a low intake of carbohydrate indefinitely is synonymous with eating higher than usual amounts of fat for a long, long time. To be able to do this, the right types of fat need to be emphasized (discussed in Chapter 16) and the individual needs to live in a supportive social and clinical sphere. If the individual is constantly told by family,

doctor, or dietitian that eating a high fat diet is dangerous, only the most curmudgeonly among us will succeed. Even if you are not convinced about the absolute safety of a well formulated low carbohydrate diet, we ask you to consider these two choices: a) remain overweight on insulin and taking two oral drugs while your fasting blood glucose remains above 200 mg/dl (11 mM) and you develop early microalbuminuria, or b) lose weight and have normal blood sugars and normal kidney function without drugs by forgoing most dietary carbohydrate long-term. What unknown risk potentially associated with the latter (i.e., a well formulated, moderate protein, high fat diet) can outweigh the likelihood of becoming a blind amputee on dialysis associated with the former?

Postscript: Clinical Details

This chapter is intended to inform the reader why a carbohydrate restricted diet is a highly effective clinical tool for the management of type-2 diabetes. It is not intended to provide instructions how to do it. That said, how to do the diet itself is well described in the authors' book *The New Atkins for a New You[5]* published in March 2010.

We have focused in this chapter on type-2 diabetes, which is primarily a disease of insulin resistance. Type-1 diabetes is physiologically very different, and this disease is not discussed here. Type-1 diabetics and some late stage type-2 individuals with very limited insulin production behave differently on a low carbohydrate diet. As a general rule, these individuals need to stay on low dose injected insulin for the duration of their carbohydrate restriction. For information on the use of carbohydrate restriction in these patients, see the excellent book by Dr. Richard K. Bernstein[2], who is himself a type-1 diabetic.

Managing the first few weeks of a low carbohydrate diet in a type-2 diabetic is a very dynamic process, particularly if the patient is taking medication for diabetic control, hypertension, or congestive heart failure. In the last century, we just admitted those patients to hospital for the initial adaptation period. In this century, we do it as outpatients using e-mail and text messaging. There is no cookie-cutter way to do this, but the key factor is open and effective 2-way communication between doctor and patient. Both need to be prepared for rapid reductions in diabetes, hypertension, and CHF medications as adaptation to the diet proceeds. As noted in Dr. Bistrian's 1976 study[120], insulin is usually withdrawn in an average of 7 days.

But the opposite is also true. If a low-carb adapted patient 'breaks the diet' by eating even transient and/or modest amounts of refined carbohydrates, all of those hard-won benefits can promptly disappear within a matter of hours and don't reappear for 3-7 days. So the withdrawn medications need to be kept close at hand, not as a sign of distrust, but as an insurance policy against the unexpected. On most days, the unused pills function as a kind of memorial to one's former drug-dependent life. But come a stress like a death in the family, a spouse bringing home the celebratory birthday cake, or winning the lottery, having the former medications in hand on Saturday night saves a trip to the ER (or perhaps a life).

For whatever reason, diabetics seem to have lots of muscle cramps. Potassium replacement if the serum value is low sometimes helps, but the true underlying cause commonly turns out to be renal magnesium wasting driven by osmotic losses. The physiology and management of this problem are discussed in Chapter 18, Pearl #9.

Chapter 16

THE IMPORTANCE OF DIETARY FAT IN LONG-TERM MAINTENANCE

Introduction

The popular use of low carbohydrate diets over the last century has been predominantly for weight loss. But as with any dietary intervention for overweight or obesity, the weight loss phase is relatively short term compared to the years and decades of reduced weight and improved health that hopefully follow. However the majority of individuals who diet to lose weight do not reach their desired goal weight, and furthermore tend to regain some of the weight they did lose within a year[43, 66, 124, 125]. Typically in these studies, a group of subjects enrolled in a randomized controlled trial reach their maximum weight loss within 6 months of starting the diet, and then begin to show weight regain by 9 or 12 months. This has prompted skeptics to brand low carbohydrate diets as useless "because no one can follow them long term". The fact that this same pattern of loss followed by regain is also seen with other calorie restricted regimens is sometimes lost on these critics.

Be that as it may, long term adherence to carbohydrate restriction is an important issue, and capturing the benefits of a low carb diet for the management of chronic conditions associated with insulin resistance requires that we address this challenge. Given the dramatic improvements in the dyslipidemia associated with metabolic syndrome and the marked improvement in diabetes management when adequate carbohydrate restriction is sustained, our purpose here is to reduce barriers to long term adherence to this type of diet.

One such barrier that is commonly perceived but seldom addressed in the research literature is how to feed the post-weight loss patient adequate energy for weight stability while maintaining the degree of carbohydrate restriction necessary to sustain the diet's benefits. Specifically, what ratio of macronutrient intake should a weight stable person eat if carbohydrates are restricted to, say, 50 grams per day? Should that person just eat more of the relatively high protein mix that was consumed during the initial weight loss phase, or does this person need to add more fat energy to achieve weight stability?

This is not a rhetorical question. Nor is it effectively addressed even by experienced low carbohydrate practitioners. Some practitioners tacitly assume that the obese person's metabolism will slow to the point that their reduced energy intake will meet daily energy needs. Others leave it to taste, appetite, and cravings to empirically lead the individual to an effective maintenance diet.

Given how poorly these 'hands off' or 'casual' approaches to low carbohydrate maintenance work in the real world, it is the purpose of this chapter to address the need for added dietary fat while keeping carbohydrates within an acceptable level of tolerance in the long-term maintenance phase of carbohydrate restriction. This is necessary for two reasons. First, the popular myth that a carbohydrate restricted diet is necessarily high in protein tends to lead the patient into added expense and sometimes dysphoria and gastro-intestinal malaise associated with too much dietary protein. Second, the demonization of fat by both consensus experts and the media has made many patients fearful of consuming the amount of fat necessary for a satisfying weight maintenance diet with the proper low-carb macronutrient balance.

Changes in Energy Intake and Expenditure Across the Diet Phases

In order to judge how best to formulate the mix of macro-nutrients in a low carbohydrate diet, it is helpful to visualize how your total energy intake will change from induction to maintenance. As indicated in the graph on the next page, a typical male with a BMI of 34 might start out eating 1600 kcal in induction while his body burns 3200 kcal per day (thus the weight loss). But after losing 50 pounds to a BMI of 27, his daily energy intake will need to increase substantially to eventually maintain him stable at that reduced weight.

Yes, when very heavy people lose a lot of weight, both their resting energy expenditure and the energy cost of 'getting around' are somewhat reduced. But then, so are the impediments (both physical and psychological) to being more active. Thus this individual might reasonably be expected to be burning 2800 kcal per day after his 50 pound loss. As an aside, the casual reader might protest that these energy expenditure numbers look pretty high. But for anyone who has worked with obese humans in a metabolic research ward, 30 kcal per kg of actual body weight in the sedentary obese and 35 kcal/kg in the post-obese moderately active adult are actually quite conservative expenditure values.

Now if our 'big loser' started out with 150 grams of protein (600 kcal) and 25 grams of carbs (100 kcal) in induction, this 700 kcal totals almost half of his intake, with the rest of the 1600 kcal (56%, or about 100 grams) coming from dietary fat. When he reaches his maintenance weight and is eating 2800 kcal/day, there is neither need nor reason for him to increase his protein intake above 150 grams, which now calculates out as 21% of his total intake. Let's also assume that he has pretty good carbohydrate tolerance, allowing him to increase that to 100 grams (400 kcal) per day. However the remainder of his daily energy intake (which now must match his expenditure) has to come from dietary fat – 1800 kcal or 200 grams per day.

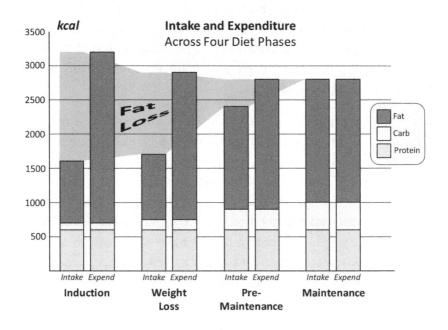

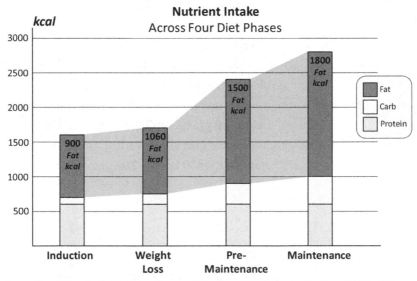

Example: Daily caloric intake and expenditure in a 5'10" man losing from 230 to 180 lbs (top) and breakdown of nutrient intake emphasizing progressive increase in fat calories (bottom). Assumes 30 kcal/kg before and 35 kcal/kg after weight loss.

"Wow", you might be saying, "that's way too much fat!"

OK, we hear you – that sounds like a lot. But what are the alternatives?

- Eat less total energy? But then our big loser will keep losing, and eventually be plagued by hunger, cravings, and low energy. The definition of 'maintenance' is that your daily energy intake equals your daily expenditure.

- Burn less energy? We want our subject to be reasonably active (not necessarily athletic), and that means burning at least 35 kcal/kg daily.

- Eat more carbohydrate? Even at 100 grams per day, our subject is 'flirting' with losing any benefits of the keto-adapted state. So adding more carbs while retaining the benefits of carbohydrate restriction is not an option. In fact, many people, particularly those who are more insulin resistant, need to eat even less carbs (e.g., 40 or 50 grams per day).

- And finally, how about more protein? Well, his 600 kcal of protein represented 38% of his energy intake during induction, but it was only 19% relative to his body's 3200 kcal expenditure. Now in maintenance when he's burning 2800 kcal per day, this 150 grams of protein equals 21% of his energy intake/expenditure. One could eat more protein than this, but there's no metabolic reason why this would be beneficial, and a variety of data indicate that too much protein causes malaise or worse (see sidebar). Even in the context of a weight maintenance very low carbohydrate diet, as the proportion of protein is increased above 30% of calories, there is a marked increase in blood urea nitrogen[126]. Fat costs less and is more satiating, and we've demonstrated that even vigorous athletes on low carb do just fine when just 15% of their energy intake comes from protein.

Human Protein Tolerance

The upper limits of human protein tolerance have not been rigorously defined. However that's not to say that this topic is completed unexplored. The Inuit knew to keep their protein intake moderate to avoid the lethargy and malaise that they knew would occur if they ate more protein than fat. Stefansson, during his year in the Bellevue experiment, was encouraged by the study investigators to eat a high protein diet for the first few weeks, causing him to be weak and sick to his stomach[11]. Finally, the Swedish investigators who developed the carbohydrate-loading hypothesis in the 1960's used lean steak as the principal food for their low-carb diets, and they had trouble keeping subjects on such a diet for more than 10 days.

Another way to examine upper limits of protein tolerance is to examine the effect of protein meals varying in amount on muscle protein synthesis. Dose response studies indicate a linear increase in skeletal muscle protein synthesis with ingestion of high quality protein up to about 20-25 grams per meal[127]. With protein intakes twice this amount, there is a marked increase in protein oxidation with no further increase in protein synthesis. When looked at over the course of a day, there is no credible evidence that protein intakes above 2.5 g/kg body weight lead to greater nitrogen balance or accumulation of lean tissue.

Another reason to avoid eating too much protein is that it has a modest insulin stimulating effect that reduces ketone production. While this effect is much less gram-for-gram than carbohydrates, higher protein intakes reduce one's keto-adaptation and thus the metabolic benefits of the diet.

As a result of these observations, plus our studies of muscle retention and function during carbohydrate restriction[27, 78, 87], we recommend daily protein intakes between 1.5 and 2.5 gram per day per kg of reference weight[5]. For a person on a weight maintaining low carbohydrate diet, this typically translates to somewhere between 15% and 25% of your daily energy intake coming from protein.

The answer to this conundrum is that our subject (and perhaps you as well) needs to make his peace with eating fat as his primary maintenance fuel. This is not a radical concept anymore. We have demonstrated how it can be safe and provide a ready and sustained fuel supply to all parts of the body. His 1800 kcal per day intake of fat is 65% of his total calories. Rest assured that an adult male can easily oxidize this amount of fat over a 24 hour period. Using indirect calorimetry in subjects adapted to low carb diets, we typically see average respiratory quotient (RQ) values well below 0.8 (even during moderate intensity endurance exercise), and this is consistent with someone burning less than 100 grams of total carbs per day, with most of the rest coming from fat.

And finally, how does this work for the typical woman? Here's the analogous graphic for a 5'6' woman who loses 30 pounds. We'll spare you the above litany of numbers for her case, but let's give her 100 grams per day of protein and 75 grams of carbohydrate and then figure out her fat intake in maintenance. Since her protein and carbs together add up to 700 kcal, to reach her 2200 kcal/day maintenance intake, she needs 1500 kcal of fat daily. With that number in your head, you will perhaps appreciate why we've included this chapter and the next one in this book.

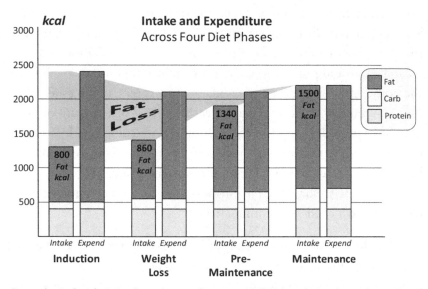

Example: Daily caloric intake and expenditure in a 5'6" woman losing from 180 to 140 lbs. Assumes 30 kcal/kg before and 35 kcal/kg after weight loss.

Dietary Fat from an Aboriginal Perspective

Given that many of our distant ancestors in non-equatorial climates ate low carbohydrate diets for at least a million years[128], it is worth considering that they may have learned useful lessons about the right mix of fat and protein by empiric observation (i.e., trial and error). This information can be gleaned from archeological observations, and also from the interaction of literate individuals with aboriginal people before their aboriginal dietary practices were irrevocably altered or replaced.

That said, however, a necessary caveat in this setting is the clear evidence for ethnocentric interpretation of aboriginal behaviors. It is a normal human tendency for us to interpret the behavior of others through the lens of our own cultural practices. Nomadic people, for example, are often viewed as unsettled or uncivilized because they do not build and maintain permanent houses or villages. As for dietary practices, people who cannot imagine themselves living without copious dietary carbohydrate will tend to look for the hidden dietary carbohydrate sources, however improbable or obscure, in the diets of hunters.

As noted in Chapter 2, we have considerable evidence that cultures evolving around hunting and herding practices selectively harvested, processed, and stored dietary fats as a weight-efficient energy source matched to their nomadic life-styles[6, 11]. As nomads, they would have had a wider range over which to hunt game (or seek pastures for their herds) than an agricultural group living at one fixed site. Thus their food supply would likely have been richer and more varied than for a village or cave-dwelling culture whose refuse heaps were more conveniently studied. So again, we repeat our warning from Chapter 2, beware of garbage dump science.

Factors Influencing Types of Fat Consumed

It's a common assumption that hunter-gatherers lived from hand to mouth, and that at any point in the annual food cycle, they were grateful for any foods they could find. While this may have been the apparent case as European incursion reduced the aboriginals' access to hunting and fishing, there is considerable evidence that pre-contact aboriginal hunters of North America actually enjoyed reasonable food security. This was accomplished through evolved cultural practices such as timing the hunt to obtain optimum carcass fat content, plus traditional food processing that preserved high fat foods to cover lean times in the hunting cycle. Examples of this mentioned above include the Inuit's autumn cache, the manufacture of pemmican, smoking and drying fatty fish (salmon, oolichan, eels), and production and storage of oolichan grease.

What this means is that for much of the year, these hunting cultures had not only a choice of how much fat they consumed, but to some degree the kind of fat as well. For example, on the North Pacific Coast, sea lions and seals could be (and were) harpooned for food and skins. And although they are rich in fat, the people of the region chose instead to focus on catching and processing the tiny oolichan as their primary fat source[12]. The reason for that is found in the chemical and physical properties of oolichan grease compared to seal oil. The latter, rich in omega-3 fats, promptly goes rancid upon exposure to air. Oolichan grease, which is low in polyunsaturates (it consists mostly of mono-unsaturated and saturated fats), is much more stable in storage, allowing it to be kept for a year or more without 'going bad'.

There is also a similar rational for pemmican, as the body fat of the buffalo, particularly in the summer, is rich in saturated fats and low in polyunsaturates, which allows the manufactured pemmican to remain solid year around, and also reduces the risk of rancidity.

But this then raises the question of the balance between desirable physical properties (solidity, low rancidity) versus the health effects of eating that fat. Perhaps these aboriginal cultures were harming themselves by eating more mono-unsaturates and saturates by avoiding sources rich in the essential polyunsaturates.

Two points mentioned previously in this book are germane to this issue. First, polyunsaturated oils rich in essential fats are important dietary constituents when one is eating a low fat diet. However if one is eating lots of fat, to get the same absolute amount of essential fats, a much smaller proportion of polyunsaturated fats (both omega-6 and omega-3) will suffice. Second, we have demonstrated in both human and animal studies that a low carb diet is associated with increased levels of essential fatty acid products (i.e., arachidonate and DHA) in blood phospholipids and tissue membranes. This occurs without signs of an increase in production, suggesting that their rate of degradation goes down when dietary carbs are limited. Thus the human requirement for essential fatty acid products may actually be somewhat reduced on an aboriginal hunting diet.

Summary

It may seem obvious, but it's important enough to reiterate that in order to preserve the therapeutic benefits from carbohydrate restriction, you have to be able live a low carbohydrate lifestyle. In other words a low carbohydrate diet does not cure insulin resistance or diabetes, but it very effectively does put it in remission. Therefore it is critical to stay at or below your unique level of carbohydrate tolerance to continue to reap these benefits long term.

When transitioning from weight loss to weight maintenance (the diet you will be eating the rest of your life), calories inevitably need to be increased. There's a lot on the line so the decision of how to do this is important. Adding carbohydrates back is a risky strategy because if you exceed your tolerance, then your previous signs and symptoms may return with a vengeance.

For those readers who play poker, adding carbs back is a bit like taking a hit in blackjack when you are holding a hard 17, 18, 19 or 20. While there is a chance you can improve your hand (i.e., you might be able to tolerate the carbs), the odds are you will bust (i.e., insulin resistance signs returns). A safer alternative is to add more fat into your diet – like having an ace in your pocket (note – we're not promoting cheating). Bottom line it's safer to stay *low carb* than to hope for a *low card*.

Chapter 17

THE JOY OF COOKING (AND EATING) FAT

Introduction:

Let go of your guilt for a second and think back. Most of us have had periods of dietary restriction after which we had free access to anything we wanted. Maybe it was a diet camp you got sent to as a teen, an extended period of intense exercise with limited food choices, or maybe just a week at your aunt's house (you know, the one who served you cold cereal with skim milk for breakfast and then spaghetti-O's and iceberg lettuce with low fat ranch dressing for supper). What was the macro-nutrient you really craved? We give you ten-to-one odds it was fat, and you probably remember just how great it tasted. No, you probably didn't sit down and eat a can of butter (see side-bar), but whether it was Ben and Jerry's ice cream, a grilled cheese sandwich, or a bacon cheeseburger, it was fat you were craving. But you probably ate it mixed with something else, unlike Joran Kropp's infamous can of butter.

In his 1996 trek to the summit of Everest after riding his bicycle there from Sweden, the adventurer Joran Kropp made three attempts to reach the summit before finally doing so. Up through the second attempt, he had been eating a vegetarian low fat diet. When he descended after his second attempt failed, he was so exhausted and depleted that he broke from his vegetarian diet and ate a large can of pure butter that he pan-handled off of the film crew that was documenting his climb. With enough fat back in his diet, on his third attempt he went on to reach the 30,030 foot summit without using supplemental oxygen.

After 50 years of demonizing fat, there are two obvious impediments to adding good fats back into our diet. The first is limited access, and the second is its preparation as foods we like to eat.

Access to fat? You ask. There's lots of fat to be had in stores and restaurants. Yes, but what kind? Most of the fat in prepared mayonnaise, dressings, sauces, and marinades is the wrong kind for a person on a high fat diet – high in polyunsaturated fat (PUFA) from the cheap, government subsidized soy, corn, and cottonseed oils used as ingredients. Olive oil is considered too expensive an ingredient by most manufacturers, and the less expensive high oleic (low PUFA) versions of safflower and sunflower oils are slow coming to market. After decades of telling consumers that high PUFA oils are good for you, it's hard for the marketing folks in the big food companies to start saying the opposite without looking foolish.

Because restricting dietary saturated fat has been a focus of nutritional recommendations since the 1970s, an unfortunate consequence has been reduced availability of the tasty and healthy traditional animal fats enjoyed by our ancestors for thousands of years. Fifty years ago, every butcher stocked lard, pork belly, and beef suet. Now a diligent shopper has to scrounge to find any of them. Duck, goose liver, beef tongue, and marrow bones were commonly eaten as gourmet foods. Now they have all but vanished from both our plates and our memories. In the past, cheese was a high fat food. Now you have to be careful when buying cheese to avoid getting the 'reduced fat' or 'low fat' options that taste like rubber or Styrofoam.

So how do we deal with this reduced access to the kinds of fat that are desirable (from both taste and health perspectives) when following a high fat, low carbohydrate diet? Clearly a key behavior is to become a careful and discriminating shopper when it comes to fat. Perhaps, as more of us ask for traditional fats, they will again become more available.

The second impediment to consuming the right kinds of fat is that we have lost the preparation skills needed to include it in our diet. Even if you did manage to buy a nice thick slab of pork belly, what would you do with it? To deal with this impediment, the rest of this chapter is devoted to selected recipes that allow you to include tasty and healthy high fat foods in your daily intake. For convenience, all of these can be made with readily available ingredients – no need to go scrounging for pork belly and/or hide your face from embarrassment when paying for it at the checkout isle.

High Fat Side Dishes

Sautéed kale with garlic and olive oil

Sadly, in modern America, kale is more often seen than eaten. It's those leaves that are stuffed between the bowls of vegetables and condiments in the typical salad bar. It is great for this because it is a pretty ruffled dark green, and it doesn't wilt for days. However when some bold individual buys it in the grocery and tries eating it, the outcome is usually grim. Why is this? And if it's so bad, why did our grandparents grow it anyway?

Kale is a member of the cabbage family, which means that it is frost-hardy and grows well in cool climates. This is actually important information. Its frost hardiness stems from its ability to shift a bit of complex sugar from its roots into its leaves when the weather turns cold. This in turn means that kale harvested in the late fall tastes sweet, in contrast to a more bitter flavor when it is harvested in summer. So the time to eat kale is in the late fall and all winter long. Let them use the summer harvest to make salad bars look appealing. Oh yes, the 'sugar' in the leaves of fall/winter kale only adds up to 3 grams of carbohydrate per half cup cooked serving, so eat it without worry about your keto-adaptation.

Ingredients:
20 or so kale leaves 6'10" long (1-2 bunches in the market)
2 cloves of garlic peeled and chopped (about 2 teaspoons)
3 tablespoons olive oil
¼ teaspoon salt

Rinse the kale in cold water and strip the flesh from the stems, tearing into postage stamp-sized pieces, allow to drain in a colander or sieve.

Brown the garlic lightly in the olive oil over medium heat in a large skillet, then add the shredded kale and salt to the hot oil and cover. Reduce the heat to simmer covered for ten minutes, stirring once or twice so it cooks evenly. Serves 3-4, 10 grams of fat per serving.

Alternative: rather than olive oil, use an ounce or two of finely chopped sow belly, fried lightly before adding the garlic. This dish can be made with collards as well.

Cucumber yogurt salad

Yogurt-based dressings are common in Greece, the Middle East, and the Indian subcontinent. Yogurt goes well with basil, dill, and lemon, allowing a variety of flavor variations. This recipe uses quite a bit of yogurt relative to the cucumbers, so the result is a bit like a cold yogurt soup with cucumber slices. And as an aside, as long as you use 'live culture yogurt', ignore the 'sugars' listed on the yogurt container's nutrition facts label. This is the amount of lactose (milk sugar) in the ingredient milk before the yogurt was made. In live culture yogurt, more than half of this is broken down to lactic acid during the fermentation process that makes yogurt. Unlike lactose, lactic acid (lactate) is easily absorbed by the body without raising your insulin level.

Ingredients:
6 medium or 4 large cucumbers peeled and sliced
4 sprigs of dill, chopped (about 2 teaspoons)

2 cups full fat plain yogurt (**not** the sweetened vanilla flavor)
2 tablespoons fresh lemon juice
2 cloves of garlic, peeled
4 tablespoons olive oil, preferably extra virgin
½ teaspoon salt
¼ teaspoon finely ground black pepper

Put the dill, garlic, olive oil, lemon juice, pepper, and salt in an 8-12 cup food processor and blend with the metal blade until smooth. Add the yogurt and blend briefly until well mixed.

Pour the yogurt mix over the cucumbers in a covered bowl and chill.

Makes 4-6 servings, each containing 12 grams of fat and 4 grams of carbohydrate.

For a nice presentation, serve in small bowls with 5-6 Belgium endive leaves as scoops.

Creamed spinach

Ingredients:
2 pounds fresh spinach
2 medium onions finely chopped
2-3 cloves of garlic finely chopped
1 cup heavy cream
2 tablespoons butter
2 tablespoons olive oil
Salt and pepper
Parmesan cheese (optional)

Wash and drain spinach and remove tough stems. In a large pot, sauté onions and garlic in butter and olive oil until translucent. Add spinach, constantly stir and press down until leaves are wilted. Add cream and cook until desired texture. Add salt and pepper to taste. Top with shaved parmesan cheese (optional).

French Fried Green Beans

Finger food to go with a steak or burger, or just by themselves for the fun of it!

Ingredients:
1 pound of fresh green beans
1 teaspoon coarse sea salt
½ teaspoon black peppercorns or rose peppercorns
¼ teaspoon garlic powder
½ teaspoon dried Italian seasoning mix
1 egg white

Pre-heat a deep fat fryer to 240°F (hot) –preferably filled with high oleic safflower oil
Rinse green beans, trim, and pat dry on a towel
Grind spices together in a mortar and pestle
Whip egg white until foamy, then coat the green beans in egg,
Put egg-coated beans in a 1-qt plastic bag and dust with ground spices, shake vigorously, and drop into hot oil. Fry for 2-3 minutes. Remove when the egg coating just starts to brown.

Tomato bisque

For those of us who grew up thinking that soup is born in a can, it's a delightful discovery how good home made soups can be, and how easy they are to make. Also, if you make your own soups from your home made broth, a serving of soup doubles as a serving of broth as well.

This recipe is best if you have ripe tomatoes and fresh basil from your garden, otherwise use plum (roma) tomatoes from the store.

Ingredients:
1 large onion sliced ¼ inch thick
6 large or 12 small tomatoes (the total volume should be 2-3 cups)
10-15 fresh basil leaves
¼ cup light olive oil
½ teaspoon finely ground black pepper
4 cups home-made chicken broth
1 cup medium (25% fat) or heavy (40% fat) cream

Rinse the tomatoes and basil leaves in cold water and drain on a towel.

Put olive oil and onions in a medium (3-4 quart) pot and brown over medium heat for about 5 minutes. The onions should end up light brown, soft, and translucent.

Cut the tomatoes in half and add them along with the basil leaves and pepper. Cover and simmer for 10 minutes, until the tomatoes are soft and cooked through.

Allow to cool for 5 minutes and place tomato/onion mixture in a food processor and blend for 60 seconds, pulsing frequently to be sure all large hunks are chopped fine.

Rinse the cooking pot, place a large sieve over it, and strain the blended tomato onion mix through it, discarding any solids that don't go thru the sieve. Depending on how smooth you want the texture of the soup, you can choose the sieve mesh size from coarse to fine.

Add the chicken broth to the tomato onion puree and warm over low heat. Heat until it just starts to steam (160-170 °F) -- don't let it boil!

Take soup off the heat and whisk in the heavy cream.

Salt to taste (the amount depends if your chicken broth was salted).

Serve warm.   Serves 6. Provides 20-25 grams fat and 5 grams carbohydrate per 10 oz serving,

Wedgie

Remember when a cheese sandwich and an iceberg lettuce wedge with ranch dressing was lunch? Now some people look back fondly at that iceberg wedge as comfort food. Well, here's a modern version, dosed with enough other stuff that it actually has measurable nutritional value.

Ingredients:
1 head of iceberg lettuce, stripped of wilted outer leaves, rinsed and drained
½ cup of crumbled blue cheese
½ cup of bacon fried lightly crisp and chopped
1 cup of sliced or diced fresh tomatoes
1 cup of sliced or diced cucumber
1 cup of yogurt blue cheese dressing (recipe below).

Slice the lettuce into quarters through the stem and remove the core from each piece.

Slice each quarter again to make equal wedges (eights) and lay the two narrow edges together in the center of a salad plate.

Arrange the toppings in the 'central valley' – for example put cucumber and tomatoes on either end and the blue cheese and bacon in the middle.

Drizzle 4 oz of the yogurt blue cheese dressing over the top when served.

Serves 4. Fat content 30 grams per serving.

High Fat, Moderate Protein, Low Carb Breakfast Smoothies

Recipes for 'low carbohydrate' smoothies abound, but most are also low in fat and assume that anything under 200 Calories from sugars qualifies as 'low carb'. Here are two basic recipes that provide enough fat and protein to keep you satisfied until lunch, and both come in at or under10 grams of carbohydrates. Note that you have your choice of sweeteners, but the argument for adding some xylitol to the mix is that it does not raise your insulin level, provides useful energy, and protects your dental health.

Also note that there are lots of different protein powders for sale, but most whey products are flavored and sweetened. Shop until you find unflavored whey powder with the lactose removed – the label should indicate about 15 grams of protein and less than one gram of carbohydrate per serving. Do not buy soy protein powder or whey/soy mix, as the soy does not dissolve well into the smoothie. This whey powder looks expensive (about $1 per 15 gram serving) but this is the same amount of protein as you get from 2 eggs.

Breakfast Berry Smoothie

Ingredients:

3 oz fresh or frozen (unsweetened) berries (strawberries, blueberries, or raspberries)
¼ cup whipping (or heavy) cream
1 tablespoon light olive oil
2 tablespoons unflavored whey protein powder (delactosed)
sweetener of choice (e.g., 1 tablespoon xylitol and 1 packet Splenda)
2-3 oz ice

Blend the ingredients at high speed until smooth (30-60 seconds)

Protein 15 grams, Fat 25-30 grams, Carbs 10 grams, Calories 330-380

Breakfast Mocca Smoothie

Ingredients:
4 oz coffee ice (frozen in ice cube tray – if frozen as a big lump in a cup or bowel, its hard to blend)
¼ cup whipping or heavy cream
1 tablespoon unsweetened cocoa powder
1 tablespoon light olive oil
2 tablespoons unflavored whey protein powder (delactosed)
sweetener of choice (e.g., 1 tablespoon xylitol and 1 packet Splenda)

Blend the ingredients at high speed until smooth (30-60 seconds)

Protein 15 grams, Fat 25-30 grams, Carbs 6 grams, Calories 310-350

<u>High Mono Dressings</u>

Yogurt blue cheese dressing

Commercial blue cheese dressings abound out there, so why should I make my own?

Answer: Better taste, better nutrition, and the right kind of fat. And if you need another reason, this recipe can be made in quantity and stored in your freezer in single serving doses. Spend 15 minutes making a batch now, and get 10 servings whenever you want them later.

Ingredients:
2 cloves of garlic,
10 fresh basil leaves
2 tablespoons fresh lemon juice
¼ cup olive oil
4 cups plain unsweetened yogurt (full or low fat, not fat-free and definitely **not** vanilla!)
8 oz crumbled blue cheese

1/8 teaspoon finely ground black pepper
1 teaspoon salt

Put the garlic, basil, lemon juice, olive oil, pepper, salt, and 4 oz (half) of the blue cheese in a blender or food processor and process until smooth. Add the yogurt and pulse until well mixed. Add the other 4 oz of blue cheese and process briefly to mix (but not blend).

Parcel out ½ cup units into snack zip-lock bags, squeezing out any extra air. Put in a container and freeze.

When needed, take individual ½ cup units out of the freezer and thaw for a few minutes in cool water.

Makes 10 half-cup servings, each containing 16 grams of fat.

Honey basil dressing

This dressing is made with real honey, but since it is mostly olive oil, the sugar content of the dressing per serving is quite low. This dressing keeps well in the refrigerator, and the roasted garlic is an excellent emulsifier, so it usually doesn't separate like most oil and vinegar concoctions.

Ingredients:
10 cloves of roasted garlic
20 fresh medium or 10 large basil leaves
¼ cup unsweetened rice vinegar (find it in the Asian foods section of your grocery)
¼ cup honey
2 packets of Splenda or 2 level tablespoons xylitol
1 cup light (not extra virgin) olive oil
½ teaspoon salt

The best way to roast garlic is to get a covered ceramic garlic roaster, slice the tops off a full garlic bulb, drizzle it with a tablespoon of olive oil and roast in the over for 45 min at 400 °F. Alternatively use a metal muffin tin, place the trimmed garlic bulb base down, drizzle with olive oil, cover each bulb with aluminum foil, and bake for 30-40 min at 400 °F. When done, the garlic cloves are soft and starting to push up out of the holes you cut in the top of each clove.

Put the roasted garlic cloves, basil leaves, rice vinegar and honey into a food processor or blender and process until very smooth (at least 2 minutes). Add the olive oil, sweetener, and salt. Blend until well mixed. Refrigerate extra in a closed container.

Makes 12 one oz servings, each containing 20 grams of fat and 5 grams of carbohydrate.

Sun-dried tomato caper dip (tapenade)

This dip is usually used on bread, but it is great with fresh vegetables, particularly Belgian endive. It is nice when made with commercial sun-dried tomatoes, but it is outrageously good when made with your own home-grown ripe tomatoes that you dry yourself.

Here's a simple way to dry tomatoes. Using a sharp knife, slice ripe tomatoes in ¼ inch thick slices blot dry on a paper towel, and lay on waxed paper in a dish in the bottom of the microwave. If you have a microwave shelf, cover it with more tomato slices as well. Run the microwave for 5 minutes at 30% power (defrost) and then for 60 minutes at 10% power. A 1000 Watt microwave puts out 100 Watts at 10% power, so it's making about as much heat as a 100 Watt light bulb, and the tomato slices should be slightly warm but not hot. Check the tomatoes after each hour, turning and rearranging as needed to help them dry evenly, repeating the same 5/60 minute heating cycle each time. This will dry 3-4 pounds of tomatoes in about 5 hrs. When done, they should be leathery in texture and still dark red. Do not dry them to black crispy wisps.

Ingredients:
3 oz of dried tomatoes (from 1.5 to 2 pounds of fresh tomatoes)
2 oz non-pareil pickled capers, lightly rinsed and drained
20 fresh basil leaves
3-5 cloves roasted garlic
1 packet Splenda or one level tablespoon xylitol
2 tablespoons unsweetened rice vinegar or wine vinegar
1 cup light olive oil

Add everything together in a food processor and blend until the tomato and basil are down to fine bits. The flavor is best if made at least an hour before serving. Remaining dip can be refrigerated for a week.

Each tablespoon contains 10 grams of fat.

Desserts

Maple walnut ice cream

Delicious, easy to make, and guilt free ice cream.

Ingredients:
½ cup English walnuts
2 tablespoons butter
2 tablespoons real maple syrup
4 cups heavy or whipping cream
2/3 cup xylitol
8 packets Splenda
2-3 drops of artificial maple flavor

Chop the walnuts to pea size. Put the nuts in a small frying pan with the butter and heat over low heat until the nuts just start to brown. Add the maple syrup to nuts and butter and stir gently over low heat until the syrup thickens and coats the nuts. Take off the heat and allow to cool. When cool, the nuts should harden into firm sticky lumps.

Mix the cream and sweeteners together and stir with a spoon until all are dissolved. Add the maple flavor and put in an ice cream maker, churning until it is thick enough to form a stable mound on a spoon. Break apart the lumps of sugary nuts and drop them into the ice cream and churn only until well distributed. Put in the freezer to firm up.

Makes 10 half-cup servings, each containing 25-40 grams of fat and 4 grams of carbs.

Blueberry cheesecake

Cheesecake would be a great source of dietary fat if it weren't for the crust and all of the sugar in it. So here's a crustless cheesecake made without any 'sugar', i.e., the stuff that raises your insulin level.

Ingredients:
2 packets plain unsweetened gelatin
1 cup xylitol (alternative ½ cup xylitol and 6 packets Splenda).
1 ½ cups water
12 oz creamed cheese
1/4 cup light olive oil
2 teaspoons vanilla extract
2 cups fresh blueberries (or sliced strawberries)

Heat the water to boiling, remove from heat and sprinkle the gelatin powder in while stirring vigorously until it is dissolved (clear).

Put the creamed cheese, olive oil, xylitol, and vanilla in a food processor, pour in the hot gelatin solution, and process until smooth.

Rinse the blueberries, pat dry, and put in the bottom of a 9-inch pie plate. Pour the still warm gelatin-cheese mix over the berries and chill in the refrigerator until it sets (30-60 min).

Makes 12 4-5 oz servings, each with 15 grams of fat and 4 grams of carbohydrate.

Alternatively, distribute the berries into 6 'snack size' Zip-Loc' bags and pour in enough cheesecake liquid to fill each bag. Squeeze out any air, seal immediately, and refrigerate). The sealed bags keep for up to a week refrigerated and a day unrefrigerated.

Summary

We hope you now have a better appreciation of how imaginative you can be with using fat to create appetizing dishes. Yes, adhering to a low carbohydrate diet does require you to give up most of those sweets and starches that once controlled you, but that's a small sacrifice when you consider what you're trading up to. Now that you are keto-adapted, using traditional fats like butter, olive oil, heavy cream, cheeses, and cream cheeses in combination with a variety of vegetable dishes are highly encouraged and part of what makes a low carbohydrate diet lifestyle enjoyable and sustainable.

Postscript: Seven Days of Low Carb Living

Here are seven days of menus one might follow on a maintenance diet providing less than 50 grams per day of total carbohydrates. The portions indicated provide between 2400 -2800 kcal per day, suitable for a normal weight, active male 5'9" tall. The division between fat, protein, and carbohydrates are listed at the bottom of each day's menu in both kilocalories and as percent of total energy.

These are not provided as a diet prescription for any one per se, but as an illustration of the amount and variety of foods one can eat on a well-formulated low carbohydrate diet. Note also that this variety is achieved while keeping the total daily carbohydrate between 30 and 50 grams. Thus someone with less carbohydrate intolerance (e.g., able to tolerate 80 grams per day) will have even an even greater variety of food choices.

Day 1 in the Low Carb Life

Breakfast
berry smoothie
(low carb, high fat)

Snacks
2 oz mixed nuts, broth
2 oz soft cheese with
6 oz celery

Lunch
2 cups mixed greens
6 oz water pack tuna
10 black olives
½ cup blue cheese
dressing (yogurt, olive oil)

Dinner
8 oz tomato bisque
8 oz steak
4 oz buttered green beans
4 oz sauteed mushrooms
4 oz maple walnut ice cream
(made w/ sucralose/xylitol)

Total: 2100 kcal fat, 600 protein, 150 carbs (74% fat, 5% carb, 21% protein)

Day 2

Breakfast
2 eggs
2 slices bacon
½ cup sauteed
mushrooms

Snacks
2 oz mixed nuts, broth
2 oz cheddar cheese

Lunch
1 cup beef broth
6 oz cold roast pork
lettuce wedge
2 oz honey basil dressing

Dinner
6 oz roast chicken with fennel
kale sauteed with bacon,
garlic, and olive oil
4 oz berries with cream

Total: 1800 kcal fat, 520 protein, 130 carbs (73% fat, 5% carb, 22% protein)

Day 3

Breakfast
black coffee
cauliflower corned-beef hash with peppers and onions (1 tbs olive oil)

Lunch
Chicken Caesar salad (takeout, 4 oz chicken)
½ packet commercial Caesar dressing (made with soybean oil)
1 tablespoon olive oil
unsweetened iced tea

Snacks
2 oz mixed nuts, broth
2 oz soft cheese with
  6 oz celery

Dinner
8 oz sorrel soup
8 oz baby back pork ribs
lettuce wedge (8 oz)
2 oz yogurt/blue cheese dressing
1 oz bacon bits
1 oz blue cheese crumbles
2 oz chopped tomatoes
2 oz chopped cucumber

Total: 1880 kcal fat, 490 protein, 120 carbs (76% fat, 5% carb, 19% protein)

Day 4

Breakfast
2-egg omelet
(1 oz each bacon, mushrooms, cheese, tomato)
black coffee

Lunch
2 cups Cobb salad (takeout)
1 tablespoon olive oil
Unsweetened iced tea

Snacks
2 oz mixed nuts, broth
10 black olives stuffed with ripe brie cheese

Dinner
8 oz French onion soup (with 2 oz guerre cheese and 2 oz onion)
Sole stuffed with creamed spinach in cheese sauce
Blueberry cheese cake

Total: 1600 kcal fat, 440 protein, 120 carbs (74 % fat, 6% carb, 20% protein)

Day 5

Breakfast
black coffee
3 oz smoked salmon
1 oz creamed cheese
1 tbsp capers
6 lettuce leaf wrappers

Lunch
2 cups mixed greens
6 oz water pack tuna
10 black olives
½ cup blue cheese
dressing (yogurt, olive oil)

Snacks
2 oz mixed nuts, broth
2 oz soft cheese with
  6 oz celery

Dinner
12 oz low carb sausage chili
8 oz grilled asparagus with
herb butter
4 oz cocoa pecan ice cream

Total: 1810 kcal fat, 530 protein, 200 carbs (71 % fat, 8% carb, 21% protein)

Day 6

Breakfast
black coffee
4 oz ham slices wrapped
around 4 oz cold grilled
buttered asparagus

Lunch
Double bacon cheeseburger
  (no bun)
Unsweetened iced tea

Snacks
2 oz mixed nuts, broth
4 oz diced cucumber, 2 oz
diced tomato
2 oz yogurt blue cheese
dressing

Dinner
8 oz bacon wrapped steak
4 oz french-fried green beans
4 oz sauteed mushrooms
4 oz maple walnut ice cream
  (made w/ sucralose/xylitol)

Total: 1755 kcal fat, 564 protein, 132 carbs (72% fat, 5% carb, 23% protein)

Day 7

Breakfast
    mocca freeze smoothie

Snacks
    2 oz mixed nuts, broth
    2 oz soft cheese with
        6 oz celery

Lunch
    2 cups mixed greens
    6 oz water pack tuna
    10 black olives
    ½ cup blue cheese
    dressing (yogurt, olive oil)

Dinner
    Coq au vin (stewed chicken)
    4 oz tomato
    4 oz sauteed mushrooms
    2 oz onion
    lettuce wedge with honey basil
    dressing

Total: 1727 kcal fat, 520 protein, 224 carbs (70% fat, 9 % carb, 21% protein)

Chapter 18

TEN CLINICAL PEARLS

One of the authors was once characterized by the statement: "Ask him directions to get to a certain bridge and he'll tell you how to build one." And perhaps there's a morsel of truth to that bit of hyperbole. We've dedicated a considerable part of this book telling you how and why low carbohydrate diets can be safe, effective, and sustainable; but as a result, some of the straightforward "what" information may have gotten lost in the clutter. So here are 10 reasonably brief take-away points (aka 'pearls') that are essential to the clinical use of carbohydrate restriction, whether for yourself or for your patient/client.

1. Honor the 'Schwatka Imperative'

This quote from Frederick Scwhatka's diary written during his epic 3000-mile trek across the Canadian Arctic in 1879-80 is the first clear description of keto-adaptation.

> "When first thrown wholly upon a diet of reindeer meat, it seems inadequate to properly nourish the system and there is an apparent weakness and inability to perform severe exertive, fatiguing journeys. But this soon passes away in the course of two to three weeks."[10]

This remarkably clear summary of the physical effects of starting on a low carbohydrate diet has been corroborated by Steve Phinney's two studies[27, 76]. And while other biochemical variables show continuing change in the adaptation process beyond 2-3 weeks, most of a person's perceived lag in intensity and stamina are eliminated sometime within this time period.

So the simple imperative is to give yourself (or so counsel your patients) 2 weeks after starting a low carb diet before beginning or increasing an exercise program or resuming a physically demanding job. And although it has not been formally studied, this same interval is required if one goes off of carbohydrate restriction (be it a week or a month) and then resumes the low carb diet. This in turn suggests that one will feel and function best if carbohydrate restriction is consistently maintained rather than followed intermittently.

2. It Only Appears to be High Protein

Most people starting out on a low carbohydrate diet intend to (and subsequently do) lose weight. This weight loss occurs because you are eating much less energy than your body is burning – typically early on up to half of your daily energy needs are coming out of your love handles. However one's protein needs (expressed as grams per day) are about the same across all phases of carbohydrate restriction, whether it's your first week in Induction or your second year in weight maintenance.

This means that your dietary protein intake is proportionately higher at the start of the diet when weight loss is occurring than later on when weight loss has stopped. Using our male example from Chapter 16, if you eat 150 grams of protein (600 Calories) in 1600 Calories per day, the diet looks to be 38% protein. Later on, when you eventually advance your energy intake to the point of achieving weight stability, say 2800 Calories per day, that same 150 grams of protein is now only 21%% of your daily energy intake. That's because in both situations most of your dietary energy needs are coming from fat. But in weight maintenance, all of this fat needs to come from your diet, so the protein content in your diet is proportionately less.

3. If You Can't Lose Your Fear of Fat, You Can't Do Low Carb Maintenance

If you had a problem metabolizing carbohydrates to start with, chances are that problem will not go away completely even after a lot of weight loss. Many people find that they get back into metabolic trouble if they add too much carbohydrate as their diet transitions into maintenance. Some people with metabolic syndrome can tolerate up to 100 grams per day of total carbs, whereas others find they need to stay under 40 to avoid the return of unhealthy blood lipids or weight regain.

But be it 40 grams or 100, that's always going to be less than 20% of your daily energy intake for a healthy active adult who burns between 1800 and 3000 Calories per day. In some cases (e.g., in a person with severe carbohydrate intolerance) carbs may total as little as 5% of dietary energy. So if protein provides 15-20% and carbs range from 5-20%, anywhere between 60% to 80% of your daily energy intake has to come from fat when you get to the point that you are maintaining your weight.

Simply put, there is no option for weight maintenance that is simultaneously low in carbohydrate and low fat. Your energy has to come from somewhere, and for people with carbohydrate intolerance, their best (and safest) long-term energy source is dietary fat. Practically speaking, that means purposefully seeking out enjoyable sources of fat and routinely including them in your diet. Given how much we've been brainwashed that fat is bad, this means patting yourself on the head, holding your hand, and telling yourself "I understand, it's OK".

Now, does this mean that you can't eat any carbs? Of course not! Whether your maintenance diet allows 40 grams or 100 gram per day of carbohydrate, you have a list of over 50 vegetables, nuts, and fruit to choose multiple servings from every day (see *The New Atkins for a New You*[5]). Our point here is that with your dietary carb intake constrained by your individual level of carbohydrate tolerance (be it 40 or 100 grams), you must get comfortable eating fat as your primary source of dietary energy if you want to succeed in low carb maintenance.

4. Be Picky About Fats

Not all fats are the same, and you need to be selective about which ones you eat for energy. On a low fat diet, because there is so little total fat intake, a fairly high proportion of what modest fat you eat needs to come from the two essential fat classes, omega-6 and omega-3. But the opposite is true when you are eating a high fat diet. There is so much omega-6 fat in our food supply that if 60% or more of your daily energy is coming from fat, it's highly unlikely you'd ever come up short. As for the omega-3's, either 3 fish meals per week or a gram of supplemental fish oil daily suffices.

It helps to think of these two essential fat classes as if they are fat soluble vitamins. While you need a modest amount of each to stay healthy, more is not necessarily better. In addition, our studies have shown that in both humans and animals adapted to low carb diets, the body makes more efficient use of both classes of essential fats compared to when fed a high carb diet.

In terms of practical choices, this implies that we give high priority to mono-unsaturates, then saturates, and make reasonable efforts to avoid rich sources of omega-6 polyunsaturates. Read labels and select foods containing olive, high-oleic safflower, and canola oils. Use olive oil or high-oleic safflower in cooking. Butter and full-fat cheese are OK, and trimming fat off of meat and skin off of poultry is no longer necessary. When possible, avoid mayonnaise and dressings made with soybean, corn, sunflower, and cottonseed oils.

5. The Salt Paradox

When the human body adapts to a low carb diet, the kidneys fundamentally change how they handle sodium. Removing most carbs from the diet causes your kidneys to aggressively secrete sodium (and along with it, extra fluid). This is why many people experience a dramatic early weight loss with carb restriction. But this means that a continuous moderate intake of sodium is necessary to keep your circulation adequate to handle 'heat stresses' like hot weather, endurance activity, or even a hot shower.

If you are eating less than 60 grams of carbohydrate per day, you need to purposefully add 2-3 grams of sodium to your daily intake (unless you are still taking diuretic medication under a doctor's direction for high blood pressure or fluid retention). And if you do hard or prolonged exercise (enough to make you sweat), one of those 'grams' needs to be consumed within the hour before you start. At or above 60 grams per day of carbs, this prescription becomes optional. However if you go out planning to exercise for 30 minutes, but find you have to stop after 15 because you feel lousy or light-headed, try it the next time with a cup of broth within an hour before exercising and see how things go.

Practically speaking, the easiest way to get this sodium is to buy standard bouillon cubes and consume 2 per day. They are cheap, compact, last months without refrigeration, and hot water is easily found. A more traditional path is to make your own meat or vegetable broth containing 1 teaspoon of salt per quart.

6. Don't Trust the Bathroom Scale With Your Mental Health

We humans are about 2/3 water. Each of us contains about 40 liters (or quarts) of the stuff, and each liter weighs a bit over 2 pounds. Our bodies effectively regulate fluid balance by adjusting urine output and sense of thirst, but this is done within a 2-liter range. Within this range, your body doesn't really care if it is up to a liter above or below its ideal fluid level.

What this means is that we all live inside a 4-pound-wide grey zone, so that from day to day we fluctuate up or down (i.e., plus or minus) 2 pounds. This happens more or less at random, so with any one weight reading you don't know where your body is within that fluid range. Your weight can be the same for 3 days in a row, and the next morning you wake up and the scale says you've 'gained' 3 pounds for no apparent reason. For people who weigh themselves frequently, this can be maddening.

There are two solutions to this problem. One, just don't weigh yourself. Or two, defeat this variability by calculating average weights. You can weigh yourself every day, and then on one day per week, calculate your average for that week (i.e., the average or mean of 7 values).

If you are really into math, you can weigh yourself every day and then each day calculate a new mean over the last 7 days. Each day you do this, you drop the oldest value and add the newest one to the calculation. And of course, for 10 bucks there's an iPhone 'App' that will do this for you (Weight Monitor by Essence Computing).

7. Exercise is a wellness tool. It is not a weight loss tool.

Most people feel better and function better if they get a modest amount of regular exercise. On average across the population, thin people get more exercise than heavy people. People who exercise regularly across a lifetime live longer. But the extrapolation of these observations – that if heavy people exercised a lot more they'd be thin and live longer – is not supported by science. Nonetheless, that is the message that many health care professionals and the media consistently communicate to heavy people.

Here are some basic (but often ignored) facts. Fitness is primarily an inherited trait. Training can increase aerobic power at most by 10-20%, but (figuratively speaking) a different choice of parents would increase or decrease your fitness by as much as 50%[129]. It takes about 350 miles of running or 1000 miles of cycling to burn off 10 pounds of body fat (assuming that your appetite doesn't increase or your metabolism slows down). Unfortunately, when heavy people exercise regularly, their resting metabolism slows – this is not a typo! – it SLOWS by 5 to 15% on average. Based on the results of 4 tightly controlled, inpatient human studies, instead of losing 10 pounds, the average person loses 7 pounds with this much exercise, and some people lose as little as 2 or 3[130-133]. These studies specifically demonstrated that this less-than-expected weight loss was attributable to the observed reduction in resting metabolic rate.

Exercise done by heavy people causes a lot of collateral damage. Think ankles, knees, hips, and low backs. So here's a radical idea (which of course is totally out of place in this book): let heavy people try carbohydrate restriction first, lose some weight (which most do without resorting to exercise), and then let them decide when to become more active once they are empowered, energized, and lighter of foot.

Making heavy people exercise is punitive. Enabling heavy people to lose weight and then become more fit is smart.

8. A Sore Muscle is a Swollen Muscle

Exercising an unfit muscle causes soreness, which is followed by improved muscle function and increased resistance of that muscle to become sore. In that sense, soreness after exercise is good (as long as it lasts less than a week and doesn't come back). Sore joints, on the other hand, are collateral damage (see above).

Most people think that if they do an intense workout (say 90 minutes of circuit training in a gym) that they should lose weight. And indeed, if you weigh before and right after such a workout, the scale goes down because of sweating and water weight loss. However, if it makes you sore for the next few days don't be surprised to see the scale go up. That's because muscle soreness indicates that your muscles are temporarily inflamed, and inflammation causes fluid retention and swelling in that muscle. Once again, don't let the scale make you crazy. Once the soreness is gone, the swelling is gone, and the scale comes back down where it's supposed to be.

9. Muscle Cramps: Unnatural Complications of a Highly Refined Diet

A distressing number of otherwise healthy people have frequent muscle cramps, and in the worst case, a muscle cramp of the heart equals sudden death. Physicians don't like to deal with muscle cramps because the only effective medication we had to stop them was banned in 1992 due to unacceptable side effects.

Muscle cramps are the end result of many contributing factors, including overuse, dehydration, and mineral inadequacies. Low serum potassium is not uncommon in people with frequent cramps, so physicians often try potassium supplements. However there is a daisy-chain leading back from muscle cramps to low blood potassium to intracellular magnesium depletion. Low carbohydrate diets don't cause muscle cramps per se (meat and leafy greens are good sources of magnesium), but neither do they miraculously get better on low carb regimens unless the underlying problem is dealt with. This is just one more reason why leafy greens and home-made broths (good sources of magnesium) are desirable components of a healthy low carb diet.

So here's the shortcut to ending most nocturnal or post-exercise muscle cramps. Take 3 slow-release magnesium tablets daily for 20 days. The proprietary brand-name product is 'Slow-Mag'®, but there are a number of equally effective generics at a fraction of the brand-name price (e.g., Mag-64® or Mag-Delay®). Most people's cramps cease within 2 weeks of starting 'Slow-Mag'®, but you should continue to take the full 20-day course (60 tabs per bottle at 3 per day lasts 20 days). If the cramps return, do it again, and then continue taking one tab per day. If the cramps return, take 2 tabs per day. Most people can be titrated to remain cramp-free by this method. Why use a more expensive slow-release magnesium preparation like Slow-Mag®? Because magnesium oxide preparations like 'milk of magnesia' cause diarrhea, passing through the small bowel before they can be effectively absorbed.

WARNING: The only contraindication to oral magnesium supplements is severe renal failure (e.g., a GFR < 30). If you have any history of kidney problems or known loss of kidney function check with your doctor before taking Slow-Mag® or its generic equivalents.

10. In Time, Your Habits Will Change

When people contemplate permanently eliminating most carbohydrate-rich foods from their diet, it often seems overwhelming. So many of our habits, both personal and social, revolve around carbohydrate foods like orange juice for breakfast and doughnuts with coffee. And some carbohydrate foods are icons of whole cultures, like bread for the French, tortillas for Mexicans, and rice for Asians. Separating yourself from these deeply ingrained behaviors is never easy.

However once an individual gets past the first few weeks of adaptation to a low carbohydrate diet, the positive changes in one's life (not just weight, but well-being and sense of empowerment) become positively reinforcing. Every day you wake up and don't have to take as much (or any) medication for diabetes, fluid retention, high blood pressure, or chronic pain is another nail in the carbohydrate coffin. Every day you stand on the scale and see that there's a lot less of you (or even that you can look past your tummy to see the number at all) is another step down your path to independence from sugars and refined carbohydrates, and towards better health and well-being.

At some point, be it months or years into the process, sticking with your low carbohydrate lifestyle is no longer a battle of intellect (I know I'm better off not eating that stuff) over desire. Eventually, it just feels right.

Section 5

GUEST CONTRIBUTORS

Chapter 19

KETOGENIC DIETS IN SEIZURE CONTROL AND NEUROLOGIC DISORDERS

by Eric Kossoff, MD
Johns Hopkins Hospital, Baltimore, Maryland

Introduction

The year was 1921. Not many years prior, neurologists had just started to realize that epilepsy was an electrical problem of the brain, not due to emotional turmoil or certainly not demonic possession. Treatments were limited to sodium bromides which could cause sexual dysfunction and phenobarbital that led to mental slowing and sedation. However, for nearly 2000 years it had been common knowledge that prolonged periods of fasting and a so-called "water diet" in the past few decades, could lead to improvement in seizures. Interestingly, even when foods were restarted after sometimes weeks, seizures would not always return. Dr. Wilder at the Mayo Clinic in Rochester, Minnesota had heard about the work of a faith healer Bernarr Macfadden and Dr. Geyelin, both of whom had used periods of starvation to help children with epilepsy. As an endocrinologist, he theorized that a high fat, low carbohydrate diet with adequate protein to maintain growth and muscle could mimic the effects of starvation. This diet, which he called the "ketogenic diet" could be continued indefinitely[134].

It was a revolution. Starting at the Mayo Clinic and spreading like wildfire, the dietary treatment of epilepsy became very popular, especially in children, many of whom had been institutionalized due to no prior effective treatments. In 1924, Dr. Peterman from the Mayo Clinic reported that the vast majority of children started on the ketogenic diet, 83%, were significantly better, with 60% completely seizure-free. Six years later, his partner Dr. Barborka used the ketogenic diet in 100 adults, with 56% showing improvement in their seizures. In the 1930s, the ketogenic diet was one of the treatments of choice for epilepsy.

Things changed in 1938. A medication called Dilantin® was invented and was touted as the "cure" for epilepsy. High fat, low carbohydrate diets were now perceived as expensive, less effective, and unnecessary. Although anticonvulsant drugs have come and gone, and sadly about a third of patients do not respond to them to treat their seizures, the ketogenic diet took a serious hit from which it has not fully recovered even to this day. Limited to select US epilepsy centers such as mine (Johns Hopkins Hospital in Baltimore), in recent decades ketogenic diets have been only used as a last resort for children with very tough epilepsy.

In November 1993, a 20-month-old boy with severe seizures named Charlie Abrahams was brought from California to Johns Hopkins Hospital to be started on the ketogenic diet by Dr. John Freeman and his dietitian, Millicent Kelly, RD. Charlie's father had to find out about the ketogenic diet in a library as it was not even mentioned as an option by his current neurologist. After only 4 days on the diet, his seizures stopped and never returned. Charlie is now 18 years old and now has been off the diet for 14 years. Needless to say, his father Jim was angry. His desire to help other families was realized through creation of the Charlie Foundation. His talent as a successful movie producer (films such as Airplane and Police Squad) prompted him to enlist the help of Meryl Streep to produce a movie, *First Do No Harm*, about a child started on the diet.

In 2010, the ketogenic diet is in a new Renaissance. It is available to my count in over 60 countries, many of whom have multiple ketogenic diet centers. There are now four ketogenic diets available: the classic ketogenic diet, the MCT (medium-chain triglyceride) diet, the modified Atkins diet (MAD), and the low-glycemic index treatment (LGIT). Ketogenic diets are being used for adults, babies, and in developing countries. No longer perceived as a treatment of last resort, they are being used first for conditions such as infantile spasms and Doose syndrome (an epilepsy syndrome in which young children suddenly develop drop seizures yet have normal intelligence).

Ketogenic diets are also being studied for use in conditions other than epilepsy, including autism, brain tumors, Alzheimer's disease, and Lou Gehrig's Disease (ALS). A 2009 expert consensus statement for optimal clinical management of children on ketogenic diets brought together 26 international experts[135]. First in 2008 in Phoenix, Arizona, then in 2010 in Edinburgh, Scotland, approximately 250 physicians, dietitians, and scientists gathered to discuss their research on dietary treatments for neurologic disorders.

Why are these diets so helpful for your brain? Basic scientists are trying to figure it out. If they can, it may open up a whole new avenue of treatments for neurologic disorders not currently available. In this chapter, the evidence of ketogenic diet therapy for brain disorders will be discussed.

The Ketogenic Diet for Epilepsy

The ketogenic diet started as a treatment for seizures and it remains by far the most common reason we use it. Studies from all over the world have consistently shown that, when used as the first treatment, about 60% of children will have at least a 50% reduction in their seizures within 6 months. Even after not responding to 3-4 different medications first, the chances of this happening are about 30%. About 1 in 10 in this drug-resistant group will become completely seizure-free, compared to half that for trying yet another drug. Given these facts, the ketogenic diet is often regarded as a very attractive option for parents.

The ketogenic diet works quickly, usually within 2 weeks. After a few days on this diet, children will start producing ketones, which can be measured at home. For decades, ketones were seen as acting like a drug, with their elevated levels being the sole reason this diet worked. However, researchers now believe the diet has favorable effects on your mitochondria (energy producing parts of your brain cells), which may be due to the high fat intake, stabilized blood glucose, or increased brain chemicals called neurotransmitters which can suppress seizures.

Clinical Case: 6 month old infant with epilepsy
(Johns Hopkins Hospital, February 2007)

CH was a 6-month-old infant who suddenly developed lightening-like jerks of her head and shoulders in clusters after naps. Increasing daily, her parents brought her to the emergency room, but no one was sure what was going on. The next day, her parents brought her back and a child neurologist saw one and diagnosed infantile spasms. In this condition, infants can suddenly develop "atonic" seizures and an electroencephalogram (EEG) filled with constant, chaotic seizure activity. It is a medical emergency due to the high likelihood (80%) of cognitive impairment if it continues.

The family was offered the two usual treatments used by child neurologists, high-dose steroids injected twice daily into the muscle, and a drug called vigabatrin. Both can be successful, but steroids can cause irritability, high blood pressure, stomach bleeds, and swelling. Vigabatrin can sometimes lead to irreversible vision damage. The parents asked for another option.

Since they came in so quickly, the ketogenic diet was offered as a 2-week trial before steroids or vigabatrin. CH's baby formula was switched to one called KetoCal® after a brief fasting period. Her last seizure was 3 days later. Two months later, her EEG normalized. Now 4 years old, CH is a completely normal, adorable little girl. Her parents have set up a foundation to promote the ketogenic diet, specifically to be offered before medications. They believe strongly parents should be given this choice.

The ketogenic diet used to treat epilepsy has some differences from the very low carbohydrate diets developed by aboriginal cultures (described in Chapter 2) and the research studies conducted by Drs. Phinney and Volek. It is higher in fat and lower in protein and carbohydrate. About 90% of the calories are derived from fat (both saturated and unsaturated), with most of the remainder (8%) protein. It is described in "ratios", with a 4:1 ratio of grams of fat vs the sum of carbohydrate and protein being the most common version. Typically started in a hospital with a 24-hour fasting period (only clear, carbohydrate-free fluids allowed), it is advanced over 4 days for the child, with the parents educated by trained dietitians on how to prepare, weigh and measure foods during that time.

The ketogenic diet seems to work slightly better for generalized seizures (coming from the entire brain all at once) than partial (focal) seizures. It works extremely well for certain types of epilepsy, including infantile spasms, Doose syndrome, tuberous sclerosis, and Dravet syndrome. In these conditions, the diet is now starting to be used sooner...even before medications if the family is interested. For children already on medications, many can have their anticonvulsant drugs reduced or even stopped, and often parents report their children as brighter and more alert. The diet is usually continued approximately 2 years and then an attempt is usually made to taper and stop the diet, after which many children remain seizure-free. However, for those whose seizures return, the diet can be resumed, and we have many children on the diet for decades due to continued seizure control benefits.

Ketogenic diets used to treat seizures do have side effects, but they are predictable, often preventable, and do not usually lead to an immediate stop to the diet. Common ones include constipation, gastroesophageal reflux, and elevations of total cholesterol and triglycerides. More rare side effects, usually preventable, are kidney stones, bone density changes, acidosis, and slowing of height gain. Multivitamins with calcium, Vitamin D, selenium, and zinc must be provided. Some children need extra carnitine as well. Weight loss does not usually occur unless the dietitian recommends that the parents limit total calories in the diet. These side effects may be more common in children due to the restrictions on their carbohydrate and protein content using these diets and their different metabolic needs.

The Modified Atkins Diet

"Alternative" diets exist, including the modified Atkins diet, often abbreviated "MAD". This diet was created in 2002 as a result of parents who observed (often on their own!) that the restrictiveness of the ketogenic diet could be lessened over time without suffering more seizures. We have since put children on this less restrictive diet from the very beginning[136].

The "modified" Atkins diet is started in the outpatient clinic (no hospital admission required), with children limiting to carbohydrates to 10 grams per day and 20 grams per day for adults. However unlike the Atkins diet, this carbohydrate restriction is not changed afterwards. Additionally, fat is strongly encouraged – we tell families the food should "shine" when a photo is taken of it. Protein, calories, and fluids are not measured; rather the parents track daily carbohydrates using carb-counting guides. This diet can be done with less cost and dietitian support, and is therefore being studied in developing countries with limited resources (e.g., Honduras and parts of India and China to name a few).

Results are similar to the ketogenic diet so far, with 78 (49%) of 160 children and adults responding. Today we recommend this alternative to the ketogenic diet mostly for teenagers, adults, and children who either cannot tolerate the level of restrictiveness of the ketogenic diet or wish to switch from the ketogenic diet after several years. In our clinic, the MAD is used in selected patients alongside the more restricted ketogenic diet, rather than as a substitute.

Another alternative to the strict ketogenic diet is the low-glycemic index treatment, created at Massachusetts General Hospital in Boston. This diet primarily watches the glycemic index (GI) of foods and recommends only carbs with a GI < 50 to minimize excursions in plasma glucose. It also seems to work!

Ketogenic diets for other neurologic disorders

Anticonvulsant drugs such as Topamax®, Neurontin®, and Lamictal® are used for many people with epilepsy around the world. However, this use is only about 1% of the total use of these drugs! How is this possible? Psychiatrists use anticonvulsants for depression, bipolar disorder, and chronic pain. Neurologists use some of these medications for migraines and neuropathy. These conditions are much more common than epilepsy by far.

Similarly, many neurologists are very interested today in the use of ketogenic diets (both the classic and modified Atkins diet) for conditions other than epilepsy[137]. Doctors in Crete have used the ketogenic diet for children with autism, and perhaps similar to reports of a gluten-free diet being helpful, so may high fat diets. Clinical trials are underway for treatment of brain tumors. Small amounts of ketones have been shown in mice to help reduce the plaques seen in Alzheimer's. There is now a human clinical trial testing if a ketogenic milkshake called Axona® results in the same benefit for people with Alzheimer's. This milkshake is available by prescription. We tested a modified Atkins diet for teenagers with severe migraines, but unfortunately many decided to stop early and it didn't appear to work well in those who stayed on it. Clinical trials are also underway for head trauma, stroke, Lou Gehrig's disease (ALS), and depression.

Clinical Case: 7 year old with autism
(Johns Hopkins Hospital, October 2004)

RA was a 6-year-old boy with autism who developed intermittent seizures at the age of 2 years. Although he had seizure control with two drugs, his parents did not like the side effects on his mood and alertness. They started the ketogenic diet at the age of 4 years and after 3 months his medications were slowly and carefully reduced and after 6 months stopped completely.

After 2 years on the ketogenic diet, our team recommended trying to come off the diet. An EEG was normal and the diet was weaned over 3-4 months. Although seizures did not return, his parents noticed an immediate increase in aggressiveness and hyperactivity once "normal" foods were restarted. With our permission, the modified Atkins diet was started, restricting carbohydrates to 10 grams per day and encouraging high fat foods. As his parents had implemented the more restrictive ketogenic diet for 2 years, this was not difficult for them to do. RA's behavior improved rapidly and he remains on the modified Atkins diet today. He likes the structure of the diet and does not cheat or ask for sugary foods.

Only time will tell which of these other neurological disorders will be responsive to the ketogenic diet and which ones will not. Researchers suspect that for certain conditions different mechanisms of action may be responsible for any observed benefit. For example, for brain tumors we may find that reduced glucose is what helps, but for Alzheimer's it may be direct effects of ketones. What is certain is that many neurologic conditions have either no cure or limited drug treatments, and ketogenic diets are certainly worth trying.

Summary

We are now at a turning point in the history of ketogenic diets for neurologic conditions. They are now back in the mainstream, widely used, and being studied in trials worldwide for both humans as well as animals to figure out how they work. No longer a last resort, they are being used in some situations before medications. We are using them for adults as well as children, conditions other than epilepsy, and in developing countries[138].

Chapter 20

THIRTY YEARS OF CLINICAL PRACTICE WITH DR. ROBERT ATKINS: KNOWLEDGE GAINED

by Jacqueline A. Eberstein, R.N.

Introduction

At the start of my career in nursing, I spent 5 years working intensive care unit and recovery room jobs in big city hospitals. After that, in 1974, I was ready to find a more stable 9 to 5 job – or so I thought. Someone talked me into going for an interview at the diet practice of Dr. Robert Atkins, whose first book was published in 1972. I hated nutrition and diet therapy in nursing school. It was boring and unimportant, and I assumed I'd have no interest in working with Dr. Atkins. The job interview was "interesting". I informed him on no uncertain terms that I had no desire to work with him; nor did I agree with his approach. He offered me the job anyway and for some unexplainable reason I accepted it. That was 1974 and I worked closely with him until I closed his medical practice six months after his death in 2003.

Like many in the medical profession, I paid very little attention to what I ate until I gained a few pounds. I had struggled with my weight since I was 12, so dieting for me was the same as for most other people; low calorie, skipping meals: being hungry on and off diets. Luckily, I had sense enough not to get into diet pills. I had a family history of diabetes and morbid obesity so I knew that I couldn't allow myself to gain too much weight before taking action.

I started work as a staff nurse in Dr. Atkins' busy practice with every intention of leaving as soon as I found something else. But to my surprise I quickly observed that his very low carbohydrate plan worked. Patients lost weight and inches easily and without hunger and cravings. Now that way of dieting appealed to me! What was also so surprising was that frequently his patients' other health complaints got better simply by changing what they ate.

Before I started working for Dr. Atkins, I had intermittent symptoms that doctors could not diagnose. After hyperthyroidism and an adrenal tumor were ruled out, all doctors could offer me were medications. One day Dr. Atkins noticed my symptoms and immediately told me to have a glucose tolerance test (GTT) at the office. He was surprised that not one doctor I saw asked me what I ate or if I had a family history of diabetes. The GTT he administered showed severe reactive hypoglycemia (RHG). At that time, one of the many criticisms of Dr. Atkins was that he diagnosed many with RHG. For this he was called a "quack". After seeing the lab results, I immediately began the Induction phase of his diet and soon felt better, just as his patients did. As long as I ate correctly and didn't skip meals I rarely experienced my prior symptoms. That remains true to this day. This was my first lesson in the power of practical nutrition (albeit outside of mainstream medical opinion). I am convinced that if I hadn't followed Dr. Atkins advice I would have had type 2 diabetes long ago. I can thank him for many things but most especially for that.

The publication of Dr. Atkins Diet Revolution in 1972 and the years since did indeed start a revolution that set off a fire-storm of sensational media, criticism, misinformation and distortion; some of which continues to this day. Fortunately, however, in the last 10 years, additional research supporting Dr. Atkins' concepts has been published. Now the Atkins plan is even presented at medical conferences as a safe, healthy and useful choice to address our ever-increasing obesity and diabetes epidemics. Perhaps because of this new research, more and more health care practitioners are now comfortable using the plan for themselves and their patients

It Began in the Medical Library

Decades ago Bob Atkins, a young doctor, found himself with an expanding belly and more than one chin. Since he had a pathological fear of hunger and loved food, he failed on low calorie diets. Out of frustration he made his way to the medical library to find a solution that he could sustain without fighting constant hunger. That quest led him to an article by Gordon et al.[139] in the October 1963 issue of *The Journal of the American Medical Association* that intrigued him. The weight loss plan he found was very similar to what would become the Atkins Diet. He followed the plan and experienced rapid, comfortable weight loss while consuming whole, nourishing, and satisfying foods.

After his own weight loss success, his first opportunity to retest the plan was while working in the medical department at AT&T. He enrolled 20 overweight executives to follow the plan for 20 weeks. They all lost weight without hunger and the follow up records show that they continued to keep it off for at least one year. The program was offered to other overweight employees and resulted in the same success. Not only did weight loss occur in relative comfort, but cholesterol values improved, subjects felt better, and common symptoms such as joint pains disappeared.

Putting It in Practice

After establishing his own internal medicine practice in New York City, Dr. Atkins fine tuned the 1963 Gordon low carb plan from JAMA, making it an important part of his practice. Word spread, especially as some New Yorkers of wealth and fame adopted the diet. It was even published as a 7 day diet plan in Vogue magazine.

After his waiting list for office appointments became much too long, someone recommended Dr. Atkins write a diet book enabling him to reach more people. In October 1972, 'Dr. Atkins' Diet Revolution' was published to instant success and immediate controversy. Remember that by the mid 1970s the "fat is bad message" was becoming the mantra of the day. Ironically, the American Medical Association was one of the most vocal critics of Dr. Atkins Diet, even though it was based on a diet he read about in JAMA, the AMA's own journal.

As chronicled in Gary Taubes' 'Good Calories, Bad Calories'[13], this unfounded criticism of Dr. Atkins continues to this day. Instead, those of us who worked with him consider him a courageous pioneer. He should be acknowledged for being a leader in pointing to the importance of stable blood sugar, insulin, triglycerides, HDL cholesterol, eggs as part of a healthy diet and for teaching us the difference between manufactured trans fats and natural fats.

After I began work at his "diet practice" in 1974 I quickly realized that he wasn't just a diet doctor – he actually practiced medicine. Admittedly, he was certainly outside of the mainstream even then. His initial patient evaluation included a 3 hour glucose tolerance test, which he later expanded to 4 then 5 hours and added fasting and postprandial insulin levels. He routinely measured triglycerides, HDL and LDL cholesterol well before these became the norm. It was by studying these results and correlating them with patient symptoms that he understood just how important controlling carbohydrate foods was to long term health. He learned a great deal from his patients. That clinical experience reinforced his belief in the importance of eating a very low carbohydrate diet consisting of unprocessed whole foods and the vast health benefits it could bring.

Dr. Atkins found that it was both the poor quality and large quantity of carbohydrate foods that provoked not only a number of chronic medical conditions but numerous day-to-day symptoms plaguing his patients. Just as a poor quality diet provoked illness, the right foods could restore health and well-being, especially in a susceptible individual. Over the years many people came to see Dr. Atkins because he and they believed that diet was a therapeutic tool. Many found answers to their health problems after the medical establishment failed them. Trusting his own clinical experience allowed him to help others regardless of the constant barrage of criticism he endured. Seeing his patients get better mattered more to him than official acceptance.

It was our clinical experience that tailoring dietary advice was especially important to our patients, most especially to those who were carbohydrate intolerant. It was extremely gratifying to see our patients' lab tests improve, their symptoms disappear, and the need for prescription medications minimized simply by using a very low carbohydrate dietary lifestyle.

The Road to Type 2 Diabetes

Dr. Atkins saw type 2 diabetes as the end result of years of 'dietary abuse', especially in those with a genetic predisposition to diabetes. He viewed it as a nutritional wear-and-tear disease. Before developing full blown diabetes, many suffer what Dr. Atkins called reactive hypoglycemia or unstable blood sugar[140]. It didn't take Dr. Atkins long to correlate an unstable blood sugar, high insulin production with weight gain, high triglycerides, low HDL cholesterol and numerous symptoms, and that this combination of symptoms followed from eating a diet containing large amounts of poor quality carbohydrates.

Surprisingly, it was not uncommon to find wide swings in blood sugar in people of normal weight, not just those with excess body fat. People with an unstable blood sugar suffer numerous symptoms that negatively affect their everyday lives. These problems resolve quickly once the optimal level of carbohydrate restriction is found. The careful assessment of glucose and insulin that Dr. Atkins did can be extremely useful to identify these individuals, but it may not be a viable choice for your patient. However, evaluating symptoms and testing their response to a very low carbohydrate diet can easily be done.

What is Unstable Blood Sugar?

Developing type 2 diabetes happens over time. Before blood sugar levels are too high, an overproduction of insulin can drop blood sugar too low. Some of the body's most prominent symptoms occur when the blood sugar is either too low or drops too quickly, setting off compensatory mechanisms to normalize blood sugar. This process results in adrenal stress and symptoms that are commonly found in our unhealthy population. People live with these symptoms every day assuming they are simply normal or part of the aging process. While these non-specific symptoms are often treated with medications, they actually result from poor dietary choices and are best diagnosed and treated by carbohydrate restriction. The dramatic difference in well-being and self-control when carbohydrates are limited implies underlying carbohydrate intolerance or addiction. Recognizing a carbohydrate intolerant patient isn't difficult!

Recognizing an Unstable Blood Sugar

Have you encountered patients with a family history of diabetes, gestational diabetes, or polycystic ovary syndrome (PCOS)? What about metabolic syndrome, an insulin resistant condition that responds well to a very low carbohydrate diet[118]? Does your patient have excessive hunger, a preoccupation with food even after eating, and an inability to control the intake of carbohydrate foods? Are symptoms relieved, at least temporarily, by eating? These are common experiences for people who are carbohydrate intolerant or addicted. Yes, carbohydrate addiction, or some may prefer to call it carbohydrate dependence, is real. The treatment is the same as for any dependence/addiction that is causing harm to the person: restrict the foods that provoke the addiction.

Common symptoms of unstable blood sugar can include any of the following.

- Mood and/or energy swings that can occur several times during the day. These can be triggers to overeat or get a quick fix from a candy bar or another high carb food.

- An increased response to stress can lead to prescription use such as tranquilizer or anti-depressant medication along with a decrease in one's ability to cope or function at an optimal level.

- Poor sleep caused by an unstable blood sugar leads to chronic sleeping pill use.

The overuse of medications is especially tragic because they are often expensive, have side effects, can make blood sugar regulation worse, and cause more weight gain as well as depleting the body of vital nutrients. Why risk putting your patient through this roller-coaster, treating symptoms with a prescription band-aid rather than practice preventive medicine by using appropriate lifestyle change? Carbohydrate restriction can address the true underlying condition, correcting these symptoms better than medication. Dr. Atkins always believed that medications were a last resort – not the first. Remember that while you are addressing the underlying cause of your patient's symptoms with carbohydrate restriction, you are also protecting their pancreatic beta-cells and preventing the onset of diabetes.

You can find a more complete list of symptoms that may indicate an unstable blood sugar in 'Dr. Atkins' New Diet Revolution', published in paperback by Avon Health, 2002, page 150. Consider having your patient complete the list before making any diet changes, and then again 4 to 6 weeks later to track progress. This is an excellent motivational tool to teach people who are carbohydrate intolerant the control they can have over their symptoms and quality of life simply by changing what they eat.

Another important observation made by Dr. Atkins was how often he saw abnormalities in postprandial blood sugar and insulin levels in patients whose fasting glucose values were close to normal. What we previously considered normal is not necessarily a safe level, as evidenced by the American Diabetes Association's recent reduction of acceptable fasting glucose from 140 to 126 mg/dl and addition of hemoglobin A1c to better discover post-prandial glucose elevations. As we learn more about blood sugar and insulin levels we are finding that even small elevations are more damaging than was first thought. Missing this finding and not making the proper dietary recommendations can mean increasing stress on beta cells and ultimately diabetes.

Is It Simply "Calories In, Calories Out"?

We hear this all the time. The more people hear it the more people believe it must be true. Similar to the phrase 'a calorie is a calorie', weight control becomes seductively simple. Except weight gain and weight loss are far more complex.

We now know a lot more about macronutrient effects on hormones and gene regulation and how these relate to fat storage and fat utilization. To continue to push the simplistic calories-in-calories-out mantra limits our therapeutic options. This is especially tragic for people who are carbohydrate intolerant. In the long run they will likely fail in making long term diet changes with a low calorie approach which is generally low in fat and high in carbohydrate. This leads to weight cycling and ultimately higher body fat. Not only is this physically damaging, but there is also the psychological cost of adding another failure, more guilt because of a lack of "will power" and lack of control.

Remember that it is easier to change behavior when what you are eating is supporting your body to work properly. That this is particularly true for people with carbohydrate intolerance was recently demonstrated by Dr. Gardner's A-to-Z Study analysis (see Chapter 7). It is up to you as their practitioner to help each patient with the best diet choice to achieve long term success based on their individual metabolic responses to food.

One Size Does Not Fit All

The one size fits all approach as demonstrated by the USDA Dietary Guidelines and the American Diabetes Association's (ADA) position that people with diabetes can eat the same foods as people without diabetes does a huge disservice to those who are carbohydrate intolerant. In essence, this position is that diabetics can eat all the carbohydrate they want; all they have to do to compensate is take more drugs.

The attitude I hear expressed at the annual International ADA conference is that most people with diabetes won't change their diets. This is an assumption that we can't afford to believe. Patients must be given unbiased access to the full range of choices, including the choice to control blood sugar by restricting both the quality and quantity of their carbohydrate intake. When given reasonable support in selecting this option, many people can and do make this change. To assume people won't or can't is simply wrong.

How much more medication and at what cost does a type-2 diabetic have to bear because of these narrow recommendations? It is well known that many people with diabetes aren't attaining their treatment goals even with intensive drug therapy. Furthermore, co-payments and treatment denials cause many people with health insurance or Medicare to skimp on testing and medications to save money.

At The Atkins Center it was almost a given that people with type 2 diabetes could reduce or eliminate their diabetic medications with a very low carbohydrate diet. This effect can be so prompt that medications often needed to be reduced from the first day to avoid drug induced hypoglycemia. Importantly, by being able to cut medication dosages, obese diabetics who have been struggling with resistance to weight loss made worse by their drugs now had the chance to succeed.

What You and Your Patients Can Expect

Most people think that all of Dr. Atkins patients came to him solely for weight management. This is far from the truth. Many overweight and obese patients presented with a litany of chronic health challenges, most caused by or exacerbated by carrying excess weight. He addressed all of their issues.

He also had considerable experience with those who appear to be at a normal, healthy weight or even underweight but ill because of poor dietary choices. Based on objective clinical testing, he knew that some people could be severely insulin resistant without being overweight. For these people he found equally good responses to an appropriate level of carbohydrate restriction.

In addition to overweight and obesity related conditions, Dr. Atkins used carbohydrate restriction to successfully treat many other health challenges including but not limited to the following: all the components of metabolic syndrome, type 2 diabetes, type 1 diabetes (reduced need for insulin and decreased hypoglycemic events), asthma, mood swings, fatigue, insomnia, depression, anxiety, headaches, migraines, allergies, inflammatory bowel syndrome, colitis, gas, bloating, GERD, joint pains, various skin eruptions including acne and psoriasis, poor memory and concentration, PCOS, and premenstrual syndrome.

Beyond Weight Loss

Dr. Atkins kept current, always carrying a medical journal and attending conferences, especially in Europe. Outside the US, he learned a great deal about non-drug therapies. He felt that medicine in the States was too drug oriented and that pharmaceuticals in many cases simply targeted symptoms and did not address the underlying cause of the illness. By the end of the 1970s he began to expand his practice using nutrients along with diet to address numerous physical complaints. The basis of his treatment was always some degree of individualized carbohydrate restriction because no amount of nutritional supplements will counter the damaging effects of a poor diet. This approach allowed him to avoid drug therapy or use lower doses for numerous disease conditions.

In many respects he was ahead of his time. For example, in the 1980s he was using fish oil supplements for inflammation and cardiovascular conditions; magnesium for heart rhythm regulation, blood pressure control and asthma; and taurine with the ketogenic phases of his diet for seizures. Well before the concept of insulin resistance syndrome and metabolic syndrome were written about, he had made the connection that dyslipidemia, glucose intolerance, and obesity clustered together and that all these markers were responsive to carbohydrate restriction. Dr. Atkins was also one of the first to talk about the negative effects of standard hormone replacement therapy and the blood sugar and weight gain side effects of a vast number of drugs.

One of the rarely talked about results of our excessive use of prescription drugs to treat lifestyle related conditions especially in an overweight population are the unwanted metabolic side effects. These include blood sugar imbalances such as hyperglycemia, hypoglycemia and weight gain. Many of the common categories of drugs prescribed today have these effects. Yet many physicians and patients are unaware of this fact. How many patients would be willing to forego another drug if it meant they could address the real cause of their symptoms and have an easier time with weight management? This is exactly why addressing lifestyle changes are needed rather than writing another Rx.

This is just the tip of the iceberg on how Dr. Atkins practiced for the last 2 decades of his life. For more information about his protocols, 'Dr. Atkins' Vita-Nutrient Solution' published in 1998 is still available today.

Dr. Atkins wanted to be remembered as a doctor of Complementary Medicine rather than a "diet doctor". This is one wish that has yet to come true. But I don't think he would be too disappointed. After all, he was a physician who strived to offer the best and safest treatment he believed he could. In the process, he helped many, and he is still doing so years after his death. Research now supports much of what Dr. Atkins observed in our clinical practice. He believed that when open-minded practitioners are given a choice of facts over dietary dogma, they will recognize that carbohydrate restriction is a practical solution to many of the health care ills of our modern way of life.

Chapter 21

A PATIENT'S PERSPECTIVE

by Jimmy Moore

Dear Doctor,

You have read about low carbohydrate diets from two well respected authorities on the topic; now let me give you the patient perspective. My name is Jimmy Moore and my story is that of a patient who took back control of his own health. I am not unlike many others who have become increasingly frustrated by the failure of conventional wisdom regarding diet and health. I had tried the recommended high-carb, low-fat diet many times over the years in my attempt to battle the bulge that had plagued me for most of my childhood and adult life. And while I experienced some transient weight loss success eating that way, one thing became abundantly clear to me – it was not a sustainable plan to meet either my nutritional requirements or to keep me satiated and happy.

I know you must be extremely frustrated by the nagging problem of heavy patients who never seem to lose weight and keep it off no matter how much you plead with them to comply with your dietary advice. But succeeding on a diet long-term is next to impossible if you are constantly plagued with hunger, cravings, irritability, and a lack of energy. The "one-size-fits-all" approach to nutrition promoted by well-meaning health organizations has been an utter and dismal failure when applied to people like me. Sadly, those of us for whom it doesn't work are left to struggle to find our own appropriate way of eating.

My first three decades of life were characterized by the extremely poor eating habits I had learned as a kid. In addition, I had acquired apathy towards being healthy because of numerous failed attempts to make that happen. In my early thirties, I found myself accepting that being fat and sick was the hand I had been dealt with no hope of ever overcoming it. It's a genuinely helpless feeling to think you will always be this way with nothing you can really do about it.

Trust me, it wasn't for a lack of trying to do all of the "right" things including trying many versions of low-fat diets, diet pills, and hours of cardiovascular exercise each week. I even took statin drugs like Lipitor® and Crestor® to help lower my cholesterol (although I experienced excruciating muscle and joint pain as a result). Like most patients, I thought the problem was me, not the presumed healthy diet I was following. In 1999 I knuckled down and started an ultra low-fat (virtually no-fat) diet. Interestingly, I did surprisingly well on it, losing around 170 pounds in just nine months. However, I literally had to will myself to be successful on this way of eating.

There was one major problem with this low-fat diet, and for me and it was a biggie–I was constantly hungry, irritable, tired, and feeling like I was losing my mind! I literally thought I was headed straight for the funny farm (I now realize the lack of fat in my diet can lead to some dubious mental side effects). My wife Christine will be the first to tell you how unpleasant I was to be around during that time. Plus, despite my weight loss success, my stomach was so bloated and big I felt like I was a lot WORSE off even though I was fitting into smaller clothes.

A month after losing all this weight Christine asked me if I would go to McDonald's and get her a chicken nuggets meal. I asked her if I could have a Big Mac® meal "just this one time." Anyone who has ever been fat knows what happened next. Frustrated by the ravenous hunger I was experiencing on my low-fat diet and refusing to live that way for the rest of my life, I binged! Not just for a few days or weeks, but for months. In just four months I regained all of my weight back and then some.

By New Year's Day in 2004, I made my way up to 410 pounds on my 6'3" body. My wife was becoming increasingly worried about my health -- for good reason. Although I didn't suffer from any major health problems at the time, my doctor had already put me on prescription medications for high cholesterol, high blood pressure and some breathing/wheezing issues. He just wrote the prescriptions and I dutifully took them. I never questioned why I was taking the drugs even when I began experiencing pain in my joints and muscles from the statin I'd been given.

In the Fall of 2003, after ripping my pants getting in my car yet again, plus a snide comment about my weight from a 6th grader, I became re-motivated to give it yet another go. But I really didn't want to feel like I did in 1999 with all the hunger, frustration, and misery associated with the low-fat diet. It was at this point in my life that I began to search for other dietary approaches that might be a better fit for my body.

My dear mother-in-law heard I wanted to try something different and she gave me a copy of *Dr. Atkins' New Diet Revolution* for Christmas that year. In the days leading up to the new year, I read the book from cover to cover. I made the fateful decision to start the Atkins diet in earnest beginning on New Year's Day 2004. This was a major turning point in my life... but of course, at the time, I was totally oblivious to just how monumental this was going to be.

It was apparent from the get-go this was going to be a challenge early on since I was so severely addicted to sugar/carbohydrate. In those first few days, I went through major carbohydrate withdrawal. After all, up to that point I'd had a 16-cans-of-Coke-a-day habit, along with eating whole boxes of Little Debbie® snack cakes (among other things). For a while, I felt like I wanted to kill myself -- I'm not kidding! The sugar withdrawal was excruciating -- perhaps as strong as someone trying to detox from crack cocaine. But thankfully I stuck with the Atkins plan because I knew I HAD to do something about my weight this time around and NOTHING was going deter me from meeting my objective.

By the end of the first month I had shed a total of 30 pounds. By the end of February, another 40 pounds were gone, and after 100 days my scale told me that 100 pounds were gone. WOW! Words simply cannot describe how I felt going through this incredible journey after so many years of recurring failure on diet after diet. At long last, I had found a plan that would work for me and I was doing it.

But wait, you might exclaim! You lost 170 pounds back in 1999. How was it different this time on a low-carb nutritional approach? Good question, because this is the best part. The key difference was that those all-too-familiar hunger pangs and the weakness that had plagued me on high-carb, low-fat diets were completely gone. Now that I was consuming a satisfyingly healthy high-fat, moderate (adequate) protein, low-carb diet, my body seemed to be "at peace" metabolically speaking. I could sense that this was the way of eating my body had been longing for all along, and now it was rewarding me for feeding it properly. I sometimes reflect on all of those years I could have been eating this way had just one insightful doctor, nutritionist, or nurse simply given me permission to do it. Yes, the Atkins diet is still considered an "outside-the-box" approach, but now you know it's a viable option that could help many of your struggling patients gain more control.

Although it wasn't an easy road by any stretch of the imagination, I am so thankful I found the healthy low-carb lifestyle because I went on to lose a total of 180 pounds on it in 2004. Writing this in 2010, I've still kept the majority of that weight off by continuing to apply low-carb principles into my daily menus. More important than my weight loss, though, was the fact that low-carb living gave me my health back. Within nine months of being on the Atkins low-carb lifestyle, all the medication I was taking became history…gone from my life forever!

To this day, I have yet to take another medication for any health ailment and I proudly tell everyone that low-carb is arguably one of the best ways to improve your health naturally without the use of drugs. Who says your health doesn't improve on the low-carb lifestyle? That's one of the main reasons why I wrote the book *21 Life Lessons From Livin' La Vida Low-*

Carb to demonstrate all of the ways low-carb works beyond weight loss. You've already learned quite a bit about that in this book as well.

Following my tremendous triple-digit weight loss in 2004, I began blogging about my experiences to encourage other patients out there that they too can lose weight and get healthy the low-carb way. In April 2005, I started the "Livin' La Vida Low-Carb" blog (http://www.livinlavidalowcarb.com/blog) as a means for educating, encouraging and inspiring others to take carbohydrate-restriction seriously when everything else had failed them. I knew from first-hand experience that it could be done and I sought to share my story in the hopes that the legacy of the late Dr. Robert C. Atkins could live on through my story.

I sincerely believe if other carbohydrate-intolerant patients like me knew they had healthy nutritional alternatives available to them, then they would enthusiastically give it a go, potentially seeing the results they have been longing for. For us as patients, support from our doctor and dietitian is invaluable when dealing with our weight and health problems, but this only 'works' if that support matches our metabolic needs. That is why the information provided in this book is so critical for medical professionals like yourselves to be exposed to.

For my part, I am privileged to have one of the most widely-read health blogs on the Internet, a Top 25 Nutrition & Fitness iTunes podcast (http://www.thelivinlowcarbshow.com/shownotes) featuring twice-weekly interviews with the world's best health experts. I have also created an online resource (http://lowcarbdoctors.blogspot.com) to help patients find medical professionals in their area who are knowledgeable and willing to support their low-carb dietary change. If you are convinced that this is a viable treatment option for your patients to try and would like to be added to this list, then I'd love to include your name and contact information to the growing number of forward-thinking doctors and nurses who realize the value of offering the low-carb lifestyle to their patients.

You possess an enormous potential to change the lives of real people who come to you for advice about how to lose weight, improve their health,

273

and become the person they have always wanted to be. Apply the principles you've learned in this book to your patients and think about my story as you are doing it. Medical professionals like you could be a part of reigniting the revolution that people like Dr. Atkins and others started many decades ago. A whole new generation of carbohydrate intolerant people are desperately looking for an alternative truth. It all revolves around healthy low-carb living and making patients feel confident about doing it for themselves. You possess the power right now to allow them to start "livin' la vida low-carb." The ball is now in your court.

Sincerely Yours,
Jimmy

Reply to Jimmy

Dear Jimmy,

We wish to thank you for your heartfelt and inspiring story, and we understand the frustration that you experienced as you struggled to find an effective low carbohydrate solution for your problem. We also appreciate the role that you have played in helping others avoid these frustrations, and yes, in inspiring others to go against the 'high carb, low fat' consensus.

As a result of your efforts and those of many other courageous individuals (see Acknowledgements, pg 277), we have a strong sense of change in attitudes and posture towards a low carbohydrate lifestyle. However the time required to significantly alter the medical consensus might be likened to an ocean liner reversing its course. Based on the escalating prevalence of obesity and metabolic syndrome, staying the course might mean we hit a proverbial iceberg. At the time of this writing, we have not 'turned the corner', so to speak. As the case of Drs. Warren and Marshall demonstrated (see pg 177), even after the definitive need for a major turn is demonstrated, the actual course correction (change in mainstream academic and clinical consensus) comes a decade later.

So when was that turn signal activated? Was it the spate of published clinical studies beginning in 2003, your experience beginning in 2004, or even later? Only time will tell. Up until that point, you will still need to patiently and firmly stand your ground against skeptics. After that point, you will proudly stand as a leader – one who by example helped us turn the corner away from the primrose path paved with sugar and starch that led many of us to obesity and its complications.

Finally, what will that change 'look like' when it happens? Will the consensus flip all the way over to the opposite view that dietary fats are good and carbs bad? We fervently hope not! Rather, if we 'stick the landing' on this paradigm shift, our flip in the consensus will leave some of us (those who are fully insulin sensitive) with the choice of continuing a high carbohydrate, low fat diet. But for those of us who have developed insulin resistance, we will finally have the unbiased option to follow a well-formulated low carbohydrate, high fat diet; allowing this major segment of humanity to recover their self-respect, well-being, and function.

We live in interesting times. May we continue to work together until that day when, walking down the street, we find that obesity is once again rare and no longer the norm.

Best Regards,
Drs. Phinney and Volek

ACKNOWLEDGEMENTS

We are blessed to be living at the right time to be able to connect the various dots that have become this book.

Almost 20 years ago, a graduate student slipped into a symposium where a professor was giving a talk about ketogenic diets. After the lecture, they conversed for a time. Five years ago, we resumed that 'conversation', from which resulted our contributions to 'The New Atkins for a New You', and now this book.

A great many generous and talented individuals have assisted us in this project. Foremost amongst these we thank Jackie Eberstein, Eric Kossoff, and Jimmy Moore for invaluable contributions that extend and complement our own experience. We thank Abby Bloch, Shelley Schlender, Graciela Anrrich, Gary Taubes, Karl and Spencer Nadolsky, Peter Defty, Anna Issakoff-Mellor, Marni Jameson, Craig Warden, Richard Seip, Carl Maresh, Laura Cusack, Laura Kunces, Brittanie Volk, Noreen Carpenter, Taryn Hand, and Richard Wood for their time and thoughtful comments on early drafts of the book.

Our current understanding of low carbohydrate diets stems from the work of many professionals extending back a hundred years or more. However being able to participate in the resurgent interest in research and clinical applications in the last decade has been both gratifying and humbling. We are honored to be included among a remarkable group of colleagues including William Kraemer, Richard Feinman, Maria Luz Fernandez, Mary Vernon, James Wortman, Douglas Bibus, Christopher Gardner, Cassandra Forsythe, Eric Westman, Gary Taubes, Donald Layman, Mary Dan and Michael Eades, and Richard K. Bernstein.

I (Steve Phinney) wish to personally thank my many teachers, mentors, and colleagues who have stimulated and guided me along the way, including: Jeff Volek, James Wortman, Richard Carpenter, Gerald Reaven, Ethan Sims, Edward Horton, Bruce Bistrian, George Blackburn, William J. Evans, Ralph Holman, Steve D. Clarke, Manabu Nakamura, Joanne Slavin, Judith Stern, Carol Stratford, and Darlene Dreon. My greatest appreciation goes to my children, Lauren and Eric, who have grown to tolerate my cooking, and to my remarkable wife Huong, without whose grasp of the 'big picture' I'd be forever lost in the details.

I (Jeff Volek) wish to personally thank many individuals who have advised and inspired me, including: Steve Phinney, William Kraemer, Maria Luz Fernandez, Richard Seip, Richard Bruno, and Richard Feinman. A special thanks to the many outstanding graduate students who have contributed to the myriad of low carbohydrate diet studies in my laboratory. Most importantly, I'm grateful for my supportive parents Jerry and Nina, my two young children-in-charge Preston (3 yr) and Reese (1 yr), and especially my extraordinary wife Ana who slows me down enough to appreciate what really matters.

ABOUT THE AUTHORS

Jeff Volek is a dietitian-scientist who has spent 15 years studying diet and exercise effects on health and performance. He has held an academic position at Ball State University and is currently an associate professor at the University of Connecticut. Dr. Volek has contributed to 3 books, 2 patents, and over 200 papers. He received his dietetic training at Michigan State University and Penrose St Francis Hospital and his PhD in Exercise Physiology from Penn State University.

Steve Phinney is a physician-scientist who has spent 35 years studying diet, exercise, fatty acids, and inflammation. He has held academic positions at the Universities of Vermont, Minnesota, and California at Davis, as well as leadership positions at Monsanto, Galileo Laboratories, and Efficas. Dr. Phinney has published over 70 papers and several patents. He received his MD from Stanford University, his PhD in Nutritional Biochemistry from MIT, and post-doctoral training at the University of Vermont and Harvard.

REFERENCES

1.   Eades, M.R. and M.D. Eades, *Protein Power: The High-Protein/Low-Carbohydrate Way to Lose Weight, Feel Fit, and Boost Your Health--in Just Weeks!* 1999: Bantam

2.   Bernstein, R.K., *Dr. Bernstein's Diabetes Solution: The Complete Guide to Achieving Normal Blood Sugars* 2007: Little, Brown and Company.

3.   *U.S. Department of Agriculture and U.S. Department of Health and Human Services. Dietary Guidelines for Americans, 2010. 7th Edition, Washington, DC: U.S. Government Printing Office, December 2010.*

4.   Reaven, G.M., *Banting lecture 1988. Role of insulin resistance in human disease.* Diabetes, 1988. 37(12): p. 1595-607.

5.   Westman, E.C., S.D. Phinney, and J.S. Volek, *The New Atkins for a New You.* 2010: Fireside.

6.   Orr, J.B. and J.L. Gilks, *Studies of nutrition: The physique and health of two African tribes* Spec. Rep. Ser. Med. Res. Coun., Lond, 1931. 155.

7.   Catlin, G., *Letters and Notes on the Manners, Customs, and Conditions of North American Indians.* Vol. 1 and 2. 1844: reprinted Dover Pubs, NY,. 1971.

8.   Stefansson, V., *The Friendly Arctic.* 1921, New York: The Macmillan co.

9.   *Rae's Arctic Correspondence 1844-1855.* 1953: Hudson's Bay Record Society.

10.   Stackpole, E.A., *The long arctic search: the narrative of lieutenant Frederick Schwatka.* 1965: The Marine Historical Society.

11.   McClellan, W.S. and E.F. Dubois, *Clinical Calorimetry. XLV: Prolonged Meat Diets with a Study of Kidney Function and Ketosis.* The Journal of Biological Chemistry 1930. 87: p. 651–668.

12.   Phinney, S.D., J.A. Wortman, and D. Bibus, *Oolichan grease: a unique marine lipid and dietary staple of the north Pacific coast.* Lipids, 2009. 44(1): p. 47-51.

13.   Taubes, G., *Good Calories, Bad Calories: Fats, Carbs, and the Controversial Science of Diet and Health* 2008: Anchor.

14.   Taubes, G., *Why We Get Fat: And What to Do About It* 2010: Knopf.

15.   *Coronary heart disease death, nonfatal acute myocardial infarction and other clinical outcomes in the Multiple Risk Factor Intervention Trial. Multiple Risk Factor Intervention Trial Research Group.* Am J Cardiol, 1986. 58(1): p. 1-13.

16.   *The Lipid Research Clinics Coronary Primary Prevention Trial results. I. Reduction in incidence of coronary heart disease.* JAMA, 1984. 251(3): p. 351-64.

17.   Atkins, R.C., *Dr. Atkins Diet Revolution.* 1972, New York: David McKay Co.

18.   *A critique of low-carbohydrate ketogenic weight reduction regimens. A review of Dr. Atkins' diet revolution.* JAMA, 1973. 224(10): p. 1415-9.

19.   [cited 2010 Dec 19]; Available from: http://www.cnpp.usda.gov/DGAs2010-DGACReport.htm.

20. Lagiou, P., et al., *Low carbohydrate-high protein diet and mortality in a cohort of Swedish women.* J Intern Med, 2007. 261(4): p. 366-74.

21. Trichopoulou, A., et al., *Low-carbohydrate-high-protein diet and long-term survival in a general population cohort.* Eur J Clin Nutr, 2007. 61(5): p. 575-81.

22. Fung, T.T., et al., *Low-carbohydrate diets and all-cause and cause-specific mortality: two cohort studies.* Ann Intern Med, 2010. 153(5): p. 289-98.

23. Phinney, S.D., et al., *The human metabolic response to chronic ketosis without caloric restriction: preservation of submaximal exercise capability with reduced carbohydrate oxidation.* Metabolism, 1983. 32(8): p. 769-76.

24. Siri-Tarino, P.W., et al., *Meta-analysis of prospective cohort studies evaluating the association of saturated fat with cardiovascular disease.* Am J Clin Nutr, 2010. 91(3): p. 535-46.

25. Yamagishi, K., et al., *Dietary intake of saturated fatty acids and mortality from cardiovascular disease in Japanese: the Japan Collaborative Cohort Study for Evaluation of Cancer Risk (JACC) Study.* Am J Clin Nutr, 2010. 92(4): p. 759-65.

26. Jakobsen, M.U., et al., *Major types of dietary fat and risk of coronary heart disease: a pooled analysis of 11 cohort studies.* Am J Clin Nutr, 2009. 89(5): p. 1425-32.

27. Phinney, S.D., et al., *The human metabolic response to chronic ketosis without caloric restriction: physical and biochemical adaptation.* Metabolism, 1983. 32(8): p. 757-68.

28. Chatham, J.C., *Lactate -- the forgotten fuel!* J Physiol, 2002. 542(Pt 2): p. 333.

29.   Forsythe, C.E., et al., *Comparison of low fat and low carbohy-drate diets on circulating fatty acid composition and markers of inflammation.* Lipids, 2008. 43(1): p. 65-77.

30.   Forsythe, C.E., et al., *Limited effect of dietary saturated fat on plasma saturated fat in the context of a low carbohydrate diet.* Lipids, 2010. 45(10): p. 947-62.

31.   Matthews, D.R., et al., *Homeostasis model assessment: insulin resistance and beta-cell function from fasting plasma glucose and insulin concentrations in man.* Diabetologia, 1985. 28(7): p. 412-9.

32.   Kannel, W.B., K. Anderson, and P.W. Wilson, *White blood cell count and cardiovascular disease. Insights from the Framingham Study.* JAMA, 1992. 267(9): p. 1253-6.

33.   Ridker, P.M., R.J. Glynn, and C.H. Hennekens, *C-reactive protein adds to the predictive value of total and HDL cholesterol in determining risk of first myocardial infarction.* Circulation, 1998. 97(20): p. 2007-11.

34.   Pradhan, A.D., et al., *C-reactive protein, interleukin 6, and risk of developing type 2 diabetes mellitus.* JAMA, 2001. 286(3): p. 327-34.

35.   Hu, F.B., et al., *Inflammatory markers and risk of developing type 2 diabetes in women.* Diabetes, 2004. 53(3): p. 693-700.

36.   Buyken, A.E., et al., *Carbohydrate nutrition and inflammatory disease mortality in older adults.* Am J Clin Nutr, 2010. 92(3): p. 634-43.

37.   Khatana, S.A., et al., *The association between C-reactive protein levels and insulin therapy in obese vs nonobese veterans with type 2 diabetes mellitus.* J Clin Hypertens (Greenwich), 2010. 12(6): p. 462-8.

38.   Borkman, M., et al., *The relation between insulin sensitivity and the fatty-acid composition of skeletal-muscle phospholipids.* N Engl J Med, 1993. 328(4): p. 238-44.

39.   Clore, J.N., et al., *Skeletal muscle phosphatidylcholine fatty acids and insulin sensitivity in normal humans.* Am J Physiol, 1998. 275(4 Pt 1): p. E665-70.

40.   Lattka, E., et al., *Do FADS genotypes enhance our knowledge about fatty acid related phenotypes?* Clin Nutr, 2010. 29(3): p. 277-87.

41.   Phinney, S.D., et al., *Obesity and weight loss alter serum polyunsaturated lipids in humans.* Am J Clin Nutr, 1991. 53(4): p. 831-8.

42.   Tang, A.B., K.Y. Nishimura, and S.D. Phinney, *Preferential reduction in adipose tissue alpha-linolenic acid (18:3 omega 3) during very low calorie dieting despite supplementation with 18:3 omega 3.* Lipids, 1993. 28(11): p. 987-93.

43.   Gardner, C.D., et al., *Comparison of the Atkins, Zone, Ornish, and LEARN diets for change in weight and related risk factors among overweight premenopausal women: the A TO Z Weight Loss Study: a randomized trial.* JAMA, 2007. 297(9): p. 969-77.

44.   Gardner, C.D., et al., *Insulin Resistance - An Effect Moderator of Weight Loss Success on High vs. Low Carbohydrate Diets.* Obesity, 2008. 16: p. S82.

45.   Boden, G., et al., *Effect of a low-carbohydrate diet on appetite, blood glucose levels, and insulin resistance in obese patients with type 2 diabetes.* Ann Intern Med, 2005. 142(6): p. 403-11.

46.   Ridker, P.M., et al., *Rosuvastatin to prevent vascular events in men and women with elevated C-reactive protein.* N Engl J Med, 2008. 359(21): p. 2195-207.

47.   Volek, J.S., M.J. Sharman, and C.E. Forsythe, *Modification of lipoproteins by very low-carbohydrate diets.* J Nutr, 2005. 135(6): p. 1339-42.

48.   de Lorgeril, M., et al., *Mediterranean diet, traditional risk factors, and the rate of cardiovascular complications after myocardial infarction: final report of the Lyon Diet Heart Study.* Circulation, 1999. 99(6): p. 779-85.

49.   Howard, B.V., et al., *Low-fat dietary pattern and risk of cardiovascular disease: the Women's Health Initiative Randomized Controlled Dietary Modification Trial.* JAMA, 2006. 295(6): p. 655-66.

50.   Lamarche, B., I. Lemieux, and J.P. Despres, *The small, dense LDL phenotype and the risk of coronary heart disease: epidemiology, patho-physiology and therapeutic aspects.* Diabetes Metab, 1999. 25(3): p. 199-211.

51.   Friedewald, W.T., R.I. Levy, and D.S. Fredrickson, *Estimation of the concentration of low-density lipoprotein cholesterol in plasma, without use of the preparative ultracentrifuge.* Clin Chem, 1972. 18(6): p. 499-502.

52.   Sniderman, A.D., et al., *Triglycerides and small dense LDL: the twin Achilles heels of the Friedewald formula.* Clin Biochem, 2003. 36(7): p. 499-504.

53.   Wang, T.Y., M. Haddad, and T.S. Wang, *Low triglyceride levels affect calculation of low-density lipoprotein cholesterol values.* Arch Pathol Lab Med, 2001. 125(3): p. 404-5.

54.   Ahmadi, S.A., et al., *The impact of low serum triglyceride on LDL-cholesterol estimation.* Arch Iran Med, 2008. 11(3): p. 318-21.

55.   McLaughlin, T., et al., *Is there a simple way to identify insulin-resistant individuals at increased risk of cardiovascular disease?* Am J Cardiol, 2005. 96(3): p. 399-404.

56.   Volek, J.S., et al., *Carbohydrate restriction has a more favorable impact on the metabolic syndrome than a low fat diet.* Lipids, 2009. 44(4): p. 297-309.

57.   Krauss, R.M., *Dietary and genetic probes of atherogenic dyslipidemia.* Arterioscler Thromb Vasc Biol, 2005. 25(11): p. 2265-72.

58.   Dreon, D.M., et al., *Low-density lipoprotein subclass patterns and lipoprotein response to a reduced-fat diet in men.* Faseb J, 1994. 8(1): p. 121-6.

59.   Dreon, D.M., et al., *A very low-fat diet is not associated with improved lipoprotein profiles in men with a predominance of large, low-density lipoproteins.* Am J Clin Nutr, 1999. 69(3): p. 411-8.

60.   Kotronen, A., et al., *Serum saturated fatty acids containing triacylglycerols are better markers of insulin resistance than total serum triacylglycerol concentrations.* Diabetologia, 2009. 52(4): p. 684-90.

61.   Miettinen, T.A., et al., *Fatty-acid composition of serum lipids predicts myocardial infarction.* Br Med J (Clin Res Ed), 1982. 285(6347): p. 993-6.

62.   Simon, J.A., et al., *Serum fatty acids and the risk of coronary heart disease.* Am J Epidemiol, 1995. 142(5): p. 469-76.

63.   Wang, L., A.R. Folsom, and J.H. Eckfeldt, *Plasma fatty acid composition and incidence of coronary heart disease in middle aged adults: the Atherosclerosis Risk in Communities (ARIC) Study.* Nutr Metab Cardiovasc Dis, 2003. 13(5): p. 256-66.

64.   King, I.B., R.N. Lemaitre, and M. Kestin, *Effect of a low-fat diet on fatty acid composition in red cells, plasma phospholipids, and cholesterol esters: investigation of a biomarker of total fat intake.* Am J Clin Nutr, 2006. 83(2): p. 227-36.

65.   Raatz, S.K., et al., *Total fat intake modifies plasma fatty acid composition in humans.* J Nutr, 2001. 131(2): p. 231-4.

66.   Shai, I., et al., *Weight loss with a low-carbohydrate, Mediterranean, or low-fat diet.* N Engl J Med, 2008. 359(3): p. 229-41.

67.   Phinney, S.D., et al., *Human subcutaneous adipose tissue shows site-specific differences in fatty acid composition.* Am J Clin Nutr, 1994. 60(5): p. 725-9.

68.   Phinney, S.D., et al., *Palmitoleate: A Biomarker of Obesity and Potential Target for Treatment* Am J Clin Nutr, 2002. 75: p. 373S.

69.   Aarsland, A. and R.R. Wolfe, *Hepatic secretion of VLDL fatty acids during stimulated lipogenesis in men.* J Lipid Res, 1998. 39(6): p. 1280-6.

70.   Wang, L., et al., *Plasma fatty acid composition and incidence of diabetes in middle-aged adults: the Atherosclerosis Risk in Communities (ARIC) Study.* Am J Clin Nutr, 2003. 78(1): p. 91-8.

71.   Lindgarde, F., B. Vessby, and B. Ahren, *Serum cholesteryl fatty acid composition and plasma glucose concentrations in Amerindian women.* Am J Clin Nutr, 2006. 84(5): p. 1009-13.

72.   Strum-Odin, R., et al., *Modification of fatty acid composition of membrane phospholipid in hepatocyte monolayer with n-3, n-6 and n-9 fatty acids and its relationship to triacylglycerol production.* Biochim Biophys Acta, 1987. 921(2): p. 378-91.

73.   Raclot, T. and R. Groscolas, *Differential mobilization of white adipose tissue fatty acids according to chain length, unsaturation, and positional isomerism.* J Lipid Res, 1993. 34(9): p. 1515-26.

74.   Garrow, J.S. and C.D. Summerbell, *Meta-analysis: effect of exercise, with or without dieting, on the body composition of overweight subjects.* Eur J Clin Nutr, 1995. 49(1): p. 1-10.

75.   Krieger, J.W., et al., *Effects of variation in protein and carbo-hydrate intake on body mass and composition during energy restriction: a meta-regression* American Journal of Clinical Nutrition, 2006. 83(2): p. 260-274.

76.   Phinney, S.D., et al., *Capacity for moderate exercise in obese subjects after adaptation to a hypocaloric, ketogenic diet.* J Clin Invest, 1980. 66(5): p. 1152-61.

77.   Young, C.M., et al., *Effect of body composition and other parameters in obese young men of carbohydrate level of reduction diet.* Am J Clin Nutr, 1971. 24(3): p. 290-6.

78.   Hoffer, L.J., et al., *Metabolic effects of very low calorie weight reduction diets.* J Clin Invest, 1984. 73(3): p. 750-8.

79.   Volek, J.S., et al., *Body composition and hormonal responses to a carbohydrate-restricted diet.* Metabolism, 2002. 51(7): p. 864-70.

80.   Volek, J.S., et al., *Comparison of energy-restricted very low-carbohydrate and low-fat diets on weight loss and body composition in overweight men and women.* Nutr Metab (Lond), 2004. 1(1): p. 13.

81.   Kraemer, W.J., et al., *Influence of exercise training on physiological and performance changes with weight loss in men.* Med Sci Sports Exerc, 1999. 31(9): p. 1320-9.

82.   Jabekk, P.T., et al., *Resistance training in overweight women on a ketogenic diet conserved lean body mass while reducing body fat.* Nutr Metab (Lond), 2010. 7: p. 17.

83.   Layman, D.K., et al., *Dietary protein and exercise have additive effects on body composition during weight loss in adult women.* J Nutr, 2005. 135(8): p. 1903-10.

84.   Volek, J.S., E.E. Quann, and C.E. Forsythe, *Low carbohydrate diets promote a more favorable body composition than low fat diets.* . Strength and Conditioning Journal, 2010. 32(1): p. 42-47.

85.   Christensen, E.H. and O. Hansen, *Arbeitsf'~ihigkeit und Ern~ihrun.* Skand. Arch. Physio, 1939. 81: p. 160-172.

86.   Bergstrom, J., et al., *Diet, muscle glycogen and physical performance.* Acta Physiol Scand, 1967. 71(2): p. 140-50.

87.   Davis, P.G. and S.D. Phinney, *Differential effects of two very low calorie diets on aerobic and anaerobic performance.* Int J Obes, 1990. 14(9): p. 779-87.

88.   McCance, R.A. and E.M. Widdowson, *Composition of the body.* Br Med Bull, 1951. 7(4): p. 297-306.

89.   Bouchard, C. and A. Tremblay, *Genetic influences on the response of body fat and fat distribution to positive and negative energy balances in human identical twins.* J Nutr, 1997. 127(5 Suppl): p. 943S-947S.

90.   Perry, G.H., et al., *Diet and the evolution of human amylase gene copy number variation.* Nat Genet, 2007. 39(10): p. 1256-60.

91.   Billings, L.K. and J.C. Florez, *The genetics of type 2 diabetes: what have we learned from GWAS?* Ann N Y Acad Sci, 2010. 1212(1): p. 59-77.

92.   Yang, M.U. and T.B. Van Itallie, *Composition of weight lost during short-term weight reduction. Metabolic responses of obese subjects to starvation and low-calorie ketogenic and non-ketogenic diets.* J Clin Invest, 1976. 58(3): p. 722-30.

93.   DeHaven, J., et al., *Nitrogen and sodium balance and sympathetic-nervous-system activity in obese subjects treated with a low-calorie protein or mixed diet.* N Engl J Med, 1980. 302(9): p. 477-82.

94.   Felig, P., *Four questions about protein diets.* N Engl J Med, 1978. 298(18): p. 1025-6.

95.   Felig, P., *Very-low-calorie protein diets.* N Engl J Med, 1984. 310(9): p. 589-91.

96.   Nansen, F., *Farthest North.* 1898, New York: Harper & Bro.

97.   Holloway, C.J., et al., *A high-fat diet impairs cardiac high-energy phosphate metabolism and cognitive function in healthy human subjects.* Am J Clin Nutr, 2011. 93(4): p. 748-55.

98.   Phinney, S.D., et al., *Normal cardiac rhythm during hypocaloric diets of varying carbohydrate content.* Arch Intern Med, 1983. 143(12): p. 2258-61.

99.   Cahill, G.F., Jr., *Starvation in man.* N Engl J Med, 1970. 282(12): p. 668-75.

100.   Huang, C.L. and E. Kuo, *Mechanism of hypokalemia in magnesium deficiency.* J Am Soc Nephrol, 2007. 18(10): p. 2649-52.

101.   Phinney, S.D., et al., *The transient hypercholesterolemia of major weight loss.* Am J Clin Nutr, 1991. 53(6): p. 1404-10.

102.   Liddle, R.A., R.B. Goldstein, and J. Saxton, *Gallstone formation during weight-reduction dieting.* Arch Intern Med, 1989. 149(8): p. 1750-3.

103.   Mozumdar, A. and G. Liguori, *Persistent increase of prevalence of metabolic syndrome among U.S. adults: NHANES III to NHANES 1999-2006.* Diabetes Care, 2011. 34(1): p. 216-9.

104.   Reaven, G.M., *Do high carbohydrate diets prevent the development or attenuate the manifestations (or both) of syndrome X? A viewpoint strongly against.* Curr Opin Lipidol, 1997. 8(1): p. 23-7.

105.   *Executive Summary of The Third Report of The National Cholesterol Education Program (NCEP) Expert Panel on Detection, Evaluation, And Treatment of High Blood Cholesterol In Adults (Adult Treatment Panel III).* JAMA, 2001. 285(19): p. 2486-97.

106.   Petersen, K.F. and G.I. Shulman, *Pathogenesis of skeletal muscle insulin resistance in type 2 diabetes mellitus.* Am J Cardiol, 2002. 90(5A): p. 11G-18G.

107.   Sonksen, P. and J. Sonksen, *Insulin: understanding its action in health and disease.* Br J Anaesth, 2000. 85(1): p. 69-79.

108.   Otero, M., et al., *Towards a pro-inflammatory and immunomodulatory emerging role of leptin.* Rheumatology (Oxford), 2006. 45(8): p. 944-50.

109.   Yang, Q., et al., *Serum retinol binding protein 4 contributes to insulin resistance in obesity and type 2 diabetes.* Nature, 2005. 436(7049): p. 356-62.

110.   Dandona, P., et al., *Metabolic syndrome: a comprehensive perspective based on interactions between obesity, diabetes, and inflammation.* Circulation, 2005. 111(11): p. 1448-54.

111.   Dhindsa, S., et al., *Differential effects of glucose and alcohol on reactive oxygen species generation and intranuclear nuclear factor-kappaB in mononuclear cells.* Metabolism, 2004. 53(3): p. 330-4.

112.   Aljada, A., et al., *Glucose ingestion induces an increase in intranuclear nuclear factor kappaB, a fall in cellular inhibitor kappaB, and an increase in tumor necrosis factor alpha messenger RNA by mononuclear cells in healthy human subjects.* Metabolism, 2006. 55(9): p. 1177-85.

113.   Seshadri, P., et al., *A randomized study comparing the effects of a low-carbohydrate diet and a conventional diet on lipoprotein*

subfractions and C-reactive protein levels in patients with severe obesity. Am J Med, 2004. 117(6): p. 398-405.

114.   Kim, J.A., et al., *Reciprocal relationships between insulin resistance and endothelial dysfunction: molecular and pathophysiological mechanisms.* Circulation, 2006. 113(15): p. 1888-904.

115.   Standaert, M.L. and R.J. Pollet, *Equilibrium model for insulin-induced receptor down-regulation. Regulation of insulin receptors in differentiated BC3H-1 myocytes.* J Biol Chem, 1984. 259(4): p. 2346-54.

116.   Knutson, V.P., et al., *Insulin resistance is mediated by a proteolytic fragment of the insulin receptor.* J Biol Chem, 1995. 270(42): p. 24972-81.

117.   Volek, J.S., et al., *Dietary carbohydrate restriction induces a unique metabolic state positively affecting atherogenic dyslipidemia, fatty acid partitioning, and metabolic syndrome.* Prog Lipid Res, 2008.

118.   Volek, J.S. and R.D. Feinman, *Carbohydrate restriction improves the features of Metabolic Syndrome. Metabolic Syndrome may be defined by the response to carbohydrate restriction.* Nutr Metab (Lond), 2005. 2: p. 31.

119.   Bantle, J.P., et al., *Nutrition recommendations and interventions for diabetes: a position statement of the American Diabetes Association.* Diabetes Care, 2008. 31 Suppl 1: p. S61-78.

120.   Bistrian, B.R., et al., *Nitrogen metabolism and insulin requirements in obese diabetic adults on a protein-sparing modified fast.* Diabetes, 1976. 25(6): p. 494-504.

121.   Gumbiner, B., J.A. Wendel, and M.P. McDermott, *Effects of diet composition and ketosis on glycemia during very-low-energy-diet therapy in obese patients with non-insulin-dependent diabetes mellitus.* Am J Clin Nutr, 1996. 63(1): p. 110-5.

122. Dashti, H.M., et al., *Ketogenic diet modifies the risk factors of heart disease in obese patients.* Nutrition, 2003. 19(10): p. 901-2.

123. Dashti, H.M., et al., *Long-term effects of a ketogenic diet in obese patients.* Exp Clin Cardiol, 2004. 9(3): p. 200-5.

124. Brehm, B.J., et al., *A randomized trial comparing a very low carbohydrate diet and a calorie-restricted low fat diet on body weight and cardiovascular risk factors in healthy women.* J Clin Endocrinol Metab, 2003. 88(4): p. 1617-23.

125. Foster, G.D., et al., *A randomized trial of a low-carbohydrate diet for obesity.* N Engl J Med, 2003. 348(21): p. 2082-90.

126. Krehl, W.A., et al., *Some metabolic changes induced by low carbohydrate diets.* Am J Clin Nutr, 1967. 20(2): p. 139-48.

127. Moore, D.R., et al., *Ingested protein dose response of muscle and albumin protein synthesis after resistance exercise in young men.* Am J Clin Nutr, 2009. 89(1): p. 161-8.

128. Parfitt, S.A., et al., *Early Pleistocene human occupation at the edge of the boreal zone in northwest Europe.* Nature, 2010. 466(7303): p. 229-33.

129. Klissouras, V., *Heritability of adaptive variation.* J Appl Physiol, 1971. 31(3): p. 338-44.

130. Bouchard, C., et al., *The response to exercise with constant energy intake in identical twins.* Obes Res, 1994. 2(5): p. 400-10.

131. Woo, R., J.S. Garrow, and F.X. Pi-Sunyer, *Voluntary food intake during prolonged exercise in obese women.* Am J Clin Nutr, 1982. 36(3): p. 478-84.

132. Phinney, S.D., et al., *Effects of aerobic exercise on energy expenditure and nitrogen balance during very low calorie dieting.* Metabolism, 1988. 37(8): p. 758-65.

133.   Heymsfield, S.B., et al., *Rate of weight loss during underfeeding: relation to level of physical activity.* Metabolism, 1989. 38(3): p. 215-23.

134.   Wilder, R.M., *The effect of ketonemia on the course of epilepsy.* Mayo Clin Bulletin 1921. 2: p. 307-308.

135.   Kossoff, E.H., et al., *Optimal clinical management of children receiving the ketogenic diet: recommendations of the International Ketogenic Diet Study Group.* Epilepsia, 2009. 50(2): p. 304-17.

136.   Kossoff, E.H. and J.L. Dorward, *The modified Atkins diet.* Epilepsia, 2008. 49 Suppl 8: p. 37-41.

137.   Baranano, K.W. and A.L. Hartman, *The ketogenic diet: uses in epilepsy and other neurologic illnesses.* Curr Treat Options Neurol, 2008. 10(6): p. 410-9.

138.   Kossoff, E.H., B.A. Zupec-Kania, and J.M. Rho, *Ketogenic diets: an update for child neurologists.* J Child Neurol, 2009. 24(8): p. 979-88.

139.   Gordon, E.S., M. Goldberg, and G.J. Chosy, *A NEW CONCEPT IN THE TREATMENT OF OBESITY.* JAMA, 1963. 186: p. 50-60.

140.   Vernon, M. and J. Eberstein, *Atkins Diabetes Revolution.* 2004: William Morrow.